DESTINY

IS WAITING ON YOU

**How to unleash your potential,
Turn your idea into reality
And achieve your dream life.**

BETTY OLOWOKERE

WHAT OTHERS ARE SAYING ABOUT
BETTY OLOWOKERE, HER STRATEGIES

Betty Olowokere is a wonderful woman who always wants to bring a significant impact on the life of everyone she comes across. She is passionate about helping people achieve their goals. She has been my strong pillar of support over the last two years.
– **Deenuka Nagrendra.**

Betty Olowokere is the Push everyone needs in their life. The dramatic change in my prayer life won't be complete without her. Her push effect has stirred up my leadership potential and dramatically changed my life. She believes in everyone. She encourages and inspires anyone who crosses her path to use their God-given gifts. She's indeed a blessing.
–**Bykota Onobrakpeya.**

This book is a lovely reminder not to take those beautiful dreams to the grave without living them out—a tool to help people push through their boundaries. –**David Ugwu**

Betty Olowokere inspires me in many ways to do more and be more. She encourages me and teaches me a lot in every area of life. Her mentoring skill is not the usual way of mentoring. She speaks with so much wisdom, not just mare wisdom but the wisdom of God. She is not only a friend but also a mentor. This book will challenge you to take hold of everything God has been saying to you.

 -Doyinsola Esther

We are spirits in mortal bodies on a different assignment. A perfect understanding of what we carry on the inside will help us manage time, resources, and energy. This book will provoke you to understand and desire to fulfill your role on earth.

–**Pastor Bode Olaleye**

DEDICATION

To everyone willing to unleash their potential and own their future.

And to my mentor,
Dean Graziosi
He made me realize that I was the help I had been waiting for all along.

Table of Contents

A MESSAGE TO YOU!

Have you heard the statement **"Que sera sera,"** which means, **"Whatever will be will be?"** I believed this statement for a long time. I watch years pass as my God given visions and ideas remain imaginations in my head. I would say to myself, I know one day. I will be this and that.

The proof of expectation is preparation. I waited for my vision, idea, and imagination to come alive without plan and action. Like many, hold onto their vision and wait for them to happen. Many wait for their lives to change one day. Life doesn't change in a day; it happens over time. Success is the result of compound actions. As much as it's desirable to dream big and imagine greatness in life, fundamental laws and principles are required to get things done. Must well understand this before your dreams become a reality.

If you continually receive a vision in the place of prayer and have a head filled with ideas and imagination of whom you have always wanted to be since childhood. This book is for you. This book is also established to guide you on essential elements required for destiny fulfillment. Many people are found in the pool of confusion with a question about where and how to start. Some people have, however, made mistakes that seemed to have threatened their destiny. This book is an eye opener on how to get back on track.

I waited so long for one day. I waited on God so long that God had to call my attention. "While you're waiting on me, I'm also waiting on you." We're partners in birthing the vision, idea, and imagination I have placed in your heart. We both have a role to play, and this is where the book's name is birthed "Destiny is waiting on you."

The moment I realize I have a role to play in my destiny, I became intentional; that was the turning point in my life. I started to take massive action, and extraordinary results became my lifestyle. Birthing your vision and idea is beyond finance. It require the cooperation of your spirit, soul, and body; it is more of inner work. The reason the chapters in this book cut across all phases of life.

If this book is all about information, you could get them anywhere else. New or more information is not what you need but a plan that work. It is time to create success habits that will help get you from where you are to where you want to be. Achieving your goal is laborious, tedious, and can even be boring, but it is worth it.

You are about to discover how to unleash your potential, achieve your goal faster, and consistently live an abundant life.

CHAPTER 1

DESTINY

The imaginations that keep coming back. The pictures that replay in your mind since childhood.

Every manufacturer once had a picture of their products in their head. They once had an imagination that kept coming back to them about the product. They are manufacturers because the pictures in their heads are now a reality. The picture that often played in their mind had simply seen the light. The manufacturer was the first to see the product before everyone else; they saw the end of the product and the purpose even before they started working on it. Nothing great happens without deep thinkers and men with grand visions. In this case, the inventions we see worldwide are simply derivatives of someone's thoughts and ideas. It takes conscious effort to make those visions a reality.

Until a product is wholly tested, it cannot be available for use. Until an architect completes the plan of a building, the building doesn't start. While the building is ongoing, the engineers in every phase of the work will keep referring back to the plan. Neglecting the plan will result in a different structure contrary to the plan. It takes an expert to draw a plan, but the unexpected happens when the engineers or the builders divert from the plan.

Before a car is manufactured, there must be considerations on various companies that will be involved in getting it done. The process may not start until there is proper consideration of some of the things needed to get the job done. However, the nature of the car to be manufactured will largely determine the necessary processes for its parts. The framework is built based on the realities in mind, transferred on paper. There must be proper information and clarity before the job can commence. Before a car is built, Different hands or technicians must be involved. You have people who build the engine. Some specialize in the wiring system, some specialize in the interior elements of the car, and others for the external features like windshield, tire, and others. All these should be considered while there must be adequate preparation before it can greet the light. The reason I said it doesn't start until a product is completed.

It's the same with you and your manufacturer. Your manufacturer knew you before you were born here on earth. Your manufacturer knew you before you were formed in your mother's womb. You were predetermined and predestinated before you showed up here on earth. Your manufacturer knows your end from the beginning. He programmed you for absolute success before you were formed and born. You do not just exist alone, the handwriting of God is upon you.

Everything you will ever need to become successful has been made available. Your manufacturer is interested in your success more than you can ever imagine. He thinks ahead of you. He's never too busy to listen to what you have to say. He is ready to guide you and journey with you here on earth. No doubt, the journey of a man on earth is never a walk in the park, and so in this process, you also have an obligation. The partnership required is between you and your manufacturer and, of course, humanity. You are a sample and proof of His love, sovereignty, and greatness, so you must not live below expectations.

As big as the planet earth is, no one; I repeat, no one has the same fingerprint as you. What does that tell you? No one is like you or will ever be like you. You are an unrepeated miracle. You are God's perfect creature. You are created perfectly for the assignment He has for you. Regardless of how you are: short, tall, light or dark, rich or poor, maybe you're a product of two races or nations like Japanese/Nigeria, raised in a polygamous family or by a single mother; God knows about it, and you are perfectly in alignment with God's plan. You're not just ordinary; you are far beyond who you think you are and people's perceptions about you. You're a mystery God daily unravel. You are that precious to your manufacturer that He handles you with care. You are made beautifully and wonderfully. You are crafted carefully. You're made from an incredible substance with great potential and simply a gift to the world.

All men are outstanding, but many have failed to see it. You tend to see otherwise due to different challenges in your life and environment. This does not rule out the truth that you're great and peculiar. Have you realized that no one can speak, dance, or write exactly like you? No one can deliver your assignment like you. You must always see yourself as the best in your field; He has chosen you because you're the best for the job. You have many skills, grace, and aptitudes that many people can covet or lust after. Still, they cannot measure up to you because they are not anointed for the same course as you, so it's a rarefied opportunity for you to be who you are and loaded in this manner. No doubt, someone somewhere might have a similar assignment, but they are not sent to the same people as you. The grace for discharge is not the same likewise the platform and system of operation. Those you're sent to will understand and connect with you deeper because you were sent to them. They just need to hear you before they get it. There is no need to fret because someone is doing something similar to you. No one can speak like you nor move like you. They don't match your energy. Every time you speak to the destinies you're connected to, they marvel like you're the only one in that field. It's just the way it is because destiny says so. You are an unrepeated miracle.

The world needs you just the way you are. In being you, you inspire yourself. In being you, you inspire us. Some people need to see you or at least hear from you and have a taste of what you carry so they can get inspired to be themselves. I mean, doing you provokes anointing and potential. This is why you have to get up and do you. You might be the one your family is waiting to see on the ladder of success. You might be the one your church, your industry, friends, colleagues, or acquaintances are waiting to see to unleash their potential. You getting up will provoke other destinies too. So, we need you to get up.

God needed to do something here on earth, and when He was done planning what He wanted to do, God made you and sent you here on earth to carry out what He needed to do, indicating that you are not here by mistake. You are not here to go to school, get married, pay bills, and die. No! You are on assignment; you are a vision in motion. You are a massive project in the hand of God, for the fact that someone calls you stupid does not make you stupid. God does not create any stupid thing. All that He created is good, and the reality of His goodness is found in you, so it behooves you to look inward and check your content, assignment, and what God wants to manufacture. You must not die until you have given all to the world and until you have fulfilled your assignment. You must not go until one and more like you have become replicated. Destiny is simply beckoning you.

To know why you're created, you must go to your manufacturer to tell you why. Only you and your manufacturer can know why you're here. Your spiritual leaders might have an idea but can't receive all the details for you; there are things God wants to tell you directly and tell only you; this is why having a relationship with your manufacturer is so important.

No one knows you like your manufacturer. If you want to know or meet you, your manufacturer is the best person to do that for you. It takes a reflection from the manufacturer's mirror to see yourself perfectly; your mind may suggest many things that may not necessarily be true. Of course, people will say a lot about you, but their opinions do not matter. What matters is an intense relationship with the one that created you, and sent you on a mission to the earth. You must stay close to His heartbeat to understand His will for your life.

The success of every product matters to the manufacturer. No product leaves the factory without being tested and trusted to carry out its functions; you were tested and trusted before you were sent here on earth. God knows you can deliver what he had placed inside of you. You don't try to become a success. You were born successful. You were born with everything you'll ever need to birth destiny. You just have to pull the trigger from here and see yourself do the magic. No demon can stop the handwriting of God, but you have to be smarter than the devil while you are determined to fulfill your course. Destiny is beckoning you.

TWO SIDES TO A DESTINY

All manufacturers produce based on good intentions in their minds. The lens you see from matters. To one person, a gun is a wrong product, while to another, a gun is a good product. To someone, an explosion is terrible, while to another, it is good. To one, someone traveling by air is terrible. To another, it is safe, faster, and perfect. Everything depends on the lens from which you see things.

In John 9:1-3, the bible tells a story of a man who was born blind. Some people around him said, "He was blind because he was a bad person. "Jesus replied, "NO," He had not sinned, and neither did his parent. He was created blind to manifest the glory of God. The lens you see your destiny from matter. This is one of the things that will determine your height in life. God had done well in creating you excellent and outstanding, but of necessity, you must see yourself through the right lens of greatness, success, and prosperity where God had created you. That is the way to become happy and become fulfilled in life. Your ability to see from the right lens will aid the fulfillment of your destiny. Remember, destiny existed before you, and you are created because someone needed to fulfill that destiny.

DESTINY AND PREPARATION

You are not designed with inferior destiny but can become inferior because of inadequate preparation. Your preparation determines the level of your manifestation. If you fail to prepare for destiny, you become rejected and unqualified.

Imagine yourself walking with closed eyes. Falling and hitting many things is inevitable for you. You might perhaps walk into your death, but when your eyes are open, you can prevent falling and hitting any element why? Because you can see and be conscious of the obstacles around you. When you are not conscious of destiny, it's like living your life with closed eyes while falling and hitting obstacles are inevitable. The first step to being better at a thing is to be aware you are not doing great in that area. Being honest with your level can be a springboard or a catalyst to drive you to excellence and perfection in the same course. This is simply one of the ways one can move forward on any course. Being conscious of destiny makes the fulfillment of destiny easy.

GOD CHOOSES DESTINY. IMPLEMENTING DESTINY WILL BE DETERMINED BY YOU.

You didn't choose your skin color, family line, nationality, temperament, and more, showing an element of destiny in you. Digging deep in the course of destiny is therefore essential. Otherwise, you may suffer a career accident if you are ignorant of the handwriting of the manufacturer. You are instrumental in fulfilling your destiny even though God has chosen it. You have to create it here on earth. If you don't create it by taking decisive action of implementing, harnessing, and establishing the course, it will remain a mirage even though it has been ordained. This is why you are said to be the creator of your destiny. **Destiny is the blueprint of the manufacturer for its products.**

DESTINY VERSUS PURPOSE:

The end of a product is considered the destiny of a product. The destiny of a washing machine is that it must wash clothes. The purpose of a washing machine is to wash clothes. You can be destined to be an author, but every book is written with different purposes and intentions. You're destined to meet some people, but each person has a different purpose to play in your life. Destiny is what will happen, the opportunity will come. Purpose is why it happens. Destiny is predetermined by divine or human will; it's usually inevitable or irresistible. Destiny is a condition where one is going to end.

PURPOSE

Purpose is the prerequisite for life. Life has no meaning without it. God will tell you about your destiny. He will share the vision of every season with you but won't tell you about the journey. God doesn't share all the details with you at once; He reveals them to you step by step. The reason being in a relationship with your Maker is highly significant. What He shows you to do is what you call dream or vision. While each vision or dream has a purpose, purpose changes in alignment with the vision/dream that God tells us to work on per season.

DREAM, VISION, AND GOAL

Dream – The pictures in your head and imaginations you can't let go of are called dream.

Vision – Those pictures are what is called vision. Vision is seeing what others can't see. Vision is different from sight. Sight focuses on the external projections while vision is seeing internally. Vision is more profound than mere sight.

Goal – These are the plans that help transforms your dreams into reality.

GIFT AND TALENT

These two words are used interchangeably; nevertheless, there is a clear difference between the two.

Gift is a natural ability, while talent is a skill developed.

INTRAPERSONAL RELATIONSHIP

An intrapersonal relationship is a relationship you have with yourself. In comparison, an interpersonal relationship is the one you have with others.

An intrapersonal relationship is a relationship with your spirit, soul, and body. We hear a lot about interpersonal relationships but not intrapersonal relationships.

THE LEVEL OF YOUR INTRAPERSONAL RELATIONSHIP WILL DETERMINE YOUR INTERPERSONAL RELATIONSHIP

To have a successful and fulfilled life, giving attention to the spirit, soul, and body is essential. All you are designed for is within you, so a clear understanding is needed in your spirit, soul, and body to understand and define yourself accurately. Knowledge is required for you to be able to see yourself the way God sees you. Understand your content profoundly, which can be discovered in the place of intimacy with your manufacturer. Hence, information that is an offshoot of wisdom, knowledge, and understanding always comes through the mind or the spirit channel. Man is original in his spirit and mind more than in his appearance and dispositions in the physical.

Men are known to be inner and outer beings. The inner being consists of two parts: the spirit and the soul. The Holy Bible makes a distinct difference in the spirit [heart] and Soul [mind]. They occupy different positions in a man while they serve separate functions. Let's see examples from the Holy Bible.

1Thessalonians 5:23 NIV. May God himself, the God of peace, sanctify you through and through. May your whole spirit, soul, and body be kept blameless at the coming of our Lord Jesus Christ. **Hebrew 4:12 NIV**. For the word of God is alive and active. Sharper than any double-edged sword, it penetrates even to dividing soul and spirit, joints and marrow; it judges the thoughts and attitudes of the heart. [The bone & marrow speaks about the body]

The writer of both scriptures makes us realize that man is tripartite, which means man exists in spirit, soul & body.

The creation of man: spirit, soul, and body
E.g., from Genesis 2:7 in the book of the Holy Bible
God made man from the dust --- body
God breathed into man ------ spirit
The man became a living soul --- soul
The meeting point of the spirit and the body birth of the soul.

When dye and water are mixed in a bowl, it results in a different entity called ink. "Dye is not ink, and neither is water ink. They are all different entities. It is the same with the spirit, soul, and body. The spirit is not soul, and neither is the soul, spirit. The spirit and the soul are different in nature but have different functions

SPIRIT, SOUL & BODY:

The spirit is the part of us that communicates with the spiritual world [God's consciousness].

The soul is the medium between the spirit and the body [self-consciousness]

The body is the part that communicates with the material world [world consciousness]. God dwells in the spirit, self-dwells in the soul & senses dwell in the body.

MAN IS A SPIRIT:

If you don't know about the law of gravity, that doesn't prevent the law from acting out on you. If you jump, the law will act, regardless of whether you are aware, like the law of electricity. If you touch a naked wire, you'll get electrocuted because being unaware of the law won't prevent you from getting electrocuted. Because you don't know you are a spirit doesn't change the fact that you are. Because you don't know that you are a spirit doesn't mean you are not participating in the spirit realm.

The spirit of man is different from the spirit of God [Holy Spirit]. Everyman has a spirit that gives them access to the spiritual world.

God communicates to us in our spirits. The soul can't receive from God. When the spirit receives from God, the soul is the medium through which the spirit communicates to the body. The spirit on its own can't act on the body without the help of the middle man, the soul.

The body also can't act in the spirit without the middle man, who is the soul. The soul stands between these two worlds, belongs to both, yet links to the spiritual world through the spirit and the material world through the body. The soul possesses the power of "Free Will." In the scripture, God refers to man as a soul because the soul expresses the individuality and personality of man. The soul is the real "I," and it's the authentic self. It's the organ in which the spirit and body merge.

God didn't make man automated. He gave you **Free will** to decide if you want to obey him or not. If the soul wishes to obey God, it allows the spirit to rule over the man, and the soul can also choose to suppress the spirit and allow the body rule.

The spirit is the noblest part of man and occupies the innermost area of the being. The body is the outermost area of the being. God intends for the spirit to rule the soul and body.

But this can be disorganized and happen the other way round, where the soul leads the body. Regardless of the part leading, the soul must give its consent. The spirit can't lead the body without the soul's consent. If the soul doesn't consent, the spirit is helpless to regulate the soul and body, but the decision is up to the soul, for therein is willpower. The power of the soul is the most substantial since both the spirit and body merge there.

THE FUNCTION OF THE SPIRIT, SOUL AND BODY

The human spirit has three functions [conscience, intuition & communion]

CONSCIENCE

Have you ever heard someone say to another person, "You don't have a conscience"? For such a statement to be uttered, it means the person has done something terrible and doesn't care or feel bad about it. When you do something terrible, and no one sees you, but it's like someone is within you judging you, that is conscience at work. It distinguishes right from wrong, not according to the mental/head knowledge.

INTUITION

Have you experience something from within telling you what was going to happen? You didn't believe it until it happened, and you were like, "'Oh! I knew this was going to happen. I just knew." People ask how you know, and all you reply is, "I don't know how, but I just knew it would happen" You need a solution to something, you've cracked your head many times and no result. You sit silently, and suddenly an idea pops up, and you shout, "Yes! That's it." You have not even tried to work out the idea you just believe it's the answer. When you put the idea into practice, it worked out. That's the intuition at work. The knowledge comes to us without help from our head knowledge. You just know. People ask how you know, and all you can say is, "I just know."

We receive all that God has to say to us through our intuition.

COMMUNION

According to John 4:24, in the Holy Bible, "God is a spirit, and those that must worship God must worship Him in spirit and truth. We commune with God in our spirits. The organ of the soul is not capable of worshiping God. The conscience judges by intuition. It condemns all conduct that does not follow the direction given by intuition.

SOUL

The soul is the authentic self. It's the seat of your personality. What makes us human belongs to the soul; emotions, mind, love, ideas and decisions all belong to the soul. Man's existence, characters, and life are all in the soul. The mind [intellect], will power [volition] & emotions are functions of the soul. This why bible reference to the soul like it's the only part of man.

EMOTION

Emotion is the expression of how you feel. You can express love, hate, anger, joy happiness. Without emotions, you become insensitive beings and can't relate to or share feelings of others.

MIND

This is the thought organ that helps you think, imagine, remember and understand. Man's intellect, reasoning, and wisdom all pertain to the mind.

The mind is the brain;

Physiologically, it addresses the brain.

Psychologically, it addresses the mind.

Lack of it makes man foolish or dull.

VOLITION (willpower)

This organ expresses your willingness or unwillingness. Without it, man is reduced to an automaton. With the knowledge of spirit, soul, and body, you realize that each has a significant role. It is essential to educate yourselves about these three parts if you want to live a victorious life.

When you are not in connection with your creator, you feel void. This is a spiritual challenge many try to solve with things like partying and having different sexual partners. It won't work. It's a spirit challenge and you can't correct by feeding your soul or body.

Some feed their spirit that they become spiritual giants while they neglect their soul. They are robust in the spirit but slim in the soul.

This shows in their intellect, emotions, and will. You can see this effect in how they talk [it reflects in their mindsets], and how they reason and do things. It reflects in their finance and other essential aspects of man.

Some feed their soul with much knowledge that they starve their spirits. This reflects in the way they do things. Without conscience, they believe they can do everything by themselves and often don't see why they need to be in a relationship with their creator.

Some feed only their body that the spirit and soul starve. You can see this in their body size, and they use words like, "I can't control the way I eat."

To experience fulfillment in life, you need to have an excellent intrapersonal relationship not with one or two parts but with the whole parts; this can give you success and fulfillment.

Spirituality is not self-development

Spirit development is educating your spirit, while self-development is educating your soul. Being healthy is taking care of your body. Hence, these three are essential for your success and fulfillment in life. Spirituality is educating yourself about the human spirit and how to communicate with the spiritual world. You have free will. So, you can decide if you want your spirit to communicate with God or demons. Herbalists, witches, wizards, and the like use their spirits to connect to the spiritual world.

Self-development is educating yourself about your mind, emotions, and will. Thus, educating your mind is so important. To become successful in any area of life including spirituality, you need to work on your mindset first. You can't get the desired result when the mindset is incorrect. Whatever message God places in your heart [spirit], you'll interpret it at the level of your mind [Soul].

To get started financially, you need to work on your mind. If you want heaven on earth marriage, you have to work on your mind because your mind is what gives you the interpretation of things. You can't get the correct result when you have wrong interpretations. Emotions are the expressions of how you feel. How you feel will determine how you relate to things. "I feel I can't do this" the moment you say that the mind will stop searching for ways to help. When you say "I can," the mind starts working on getting information to help you out. When the mind is clear about what you want, it searches the spirit and the soul for answers.

HEALTHY BODY

You need a healthy body to carry out the command the body receive from your spirit and soul. The body needs to be healthy to birth destiny. The body needs to be healthy to be the best version of yourself. Your body needs to be healthy to express what's happening inside you. Imagine someone is happy but can't smile or jump because they are down with a sickness.

A man can be successful and not be fulfilled. You have heard about many wealthy people who have committed suicide. They are successful, but their pain finds a way to make them believe there is no reason to continue living. But a man in alignment with destiny and implementing visions will have a firm conviction of why they live. They rarely think of suicide. Fulfilling destiny gives a sense of I have a reason to live. Fulfillment is that internal joy you experience when you do something that impacts others. The stylish smile from within brings joy.

FREE WILL

Though destiny is determined, you have free will with which you can choose to fulfill destiny or not.

Every man has free will. Free will is your ability to choose to live free or enslaved, do good or bad. Some use their free will, while others make excuses for not using their free will. No one can enslave you unless you permit them.

A MAN'S WILL

This organ is for decision making. The ability to make choices, and acting at one's discretion.

A man's will is his authentic self. When you say "I want, or I decide." it's your will that wants and decides. Your emotions express how you feel. Your mind tells you what to think. Your **WILL** communicates what you want. The **will** is the most influential component of your entire being. The **will** is more profound than emotions and the mind.

The primary purpose of religion is to have a relationship with God, so your **will** can align with God's **will**. God will never force you to do his **will.**

FULFILLMENT OF DESTINY

God doesn't go against your **will**. If He wants you to do something, He shares the vision with you, and when you don't get it, He exposes you to teachings and books and sends people to you. Sometimes, He may put you in a situation to challenge your minds to see differently and help you understand the vision He had shared with you. God will never force you to do His will. **To fulfill destiny, you have to partner with God intentionally.** God decides and ordains your destiny, but you'll decide if it will be fulfilled here on earth or not. As you fellowship and walk with God, He guides you to walk in alignment with destiny. As you commune with Him, He tells you the steps to take. Destiny can wait forever if you refuse to get up and do something about it. But God has programmed you in a way destiny comes knocking and keeps coming back throughout a man's life.

You are conscious of who you want to be when you are little. As you grow up seeing challenges and facing them, you let go of those dreams because your big selves consider them impossible or difficult to accomplish.

Don't forget the pictures of who you want to become. The imaginations you can't let go of. It is destiny calling your attention. Give your all to make it a reality. Be courageous to chase after those pictures in your head. They are real. It's your creator speaking to you. While you're waiting for things to change, God is waiting on you to change things. While you're waiting on destiny,

destiny is waiting for you to get up and take massive action towards the pictures and the imaginations you can't let go.

CHAPTER 2

JOURNEY OF DISCOVERY

"The greatest discovery in life is self-discovery. Until you find yourself you will always be someone else. Become yourself."

- Myles Munroe.

Discovery is intentional!

"Discovery is an act of finding out or learning for the first time" - Merriam Webster,

Self-discovery is a life journey. As long as you live, you will continue to meet a new version of yourself. Either you are conscious about discovering your new self or get stuck in the old version of you. The journey of discovery is intentional, not easy, but it is always worth it. It's never a straight road but a bumpy and undulating one.

The worst thing that can ever happen to a man is to lose his true nature, definition, and understanding of himself. If you fail to realize this truth, many people will tag you with different nomenclature contrary to your real identity. They will simply submit their resolutions about you, and you would assume that is who you are without apology. The journey, however, will not be a walk in the park, but after persistent effort has been made, it will yield a diamond and give you the best definition of yourself.

Your creator has been speaking who you were created to be since you were a child. I'm sure you have voiced out who you were created to be multiple times when you were a child. When you were young, you have fewer things to be concerned about, the internal world was more real than the external world. You express yourselves and allow your creative value to find expression. As you grow older, you get carried away by life challenges. The external world becomes more real than the inner World. This suppresses the voice and expression of your authentic self from within. The challenges make you believe it is difficult for those pictures in your head to become a reality. So you start acting small and ignore those pictures. They might be suppressed, they still resurface when your mind is quiet.

The journey to self-discovery is personal, and intentional. You can decide to listen to your inner man or ignore. Each action taken simply has consequences. Imagine how awful will it be for a man to have a diamond crying for attention inside of him while he goes about the street begging for bread.

Man on the physical is full of deception. Your eyes simply makes you believe that everything it sees is precisely the way it is. But this is not true. Many beautiful things in the open are nothing but a mess on the inside. It is, therefore, not all about the physical. One can be presented with his best meal, sumptuous and delicious but poisoned. Of course, the food smelled good and was quite delicious but poisoned. This is to show that many things can be beautiful but not good. There are a lot of beautiful buildings that simply collapsed, and this is a result of a faulty foundation. Learn to switch to your inside to find the truth, and you will also find a better version of yourself and a right understanding of who you are and your purpose in life.

INTERNAL GPS:
The Intellect has little to do with the road to discovery. There comes a leap in consciousness, call it INTUITION or what you will, and the solution will come to you, and you don't know how or why. All great discoveries are made in this way. ---- Albert Einstein.

From the quote above,
Albert said, **"Solutions come to you, and you don't know how or why."**
How can man get solution from within? There has to be a genius inside of you that communicates to you.

Albert and Many people have gotten solution while sleeping. I have listened to testimonies of people receiving solutions by hearing from within. I'm also a testimony. Many times I have received answers from within. The truth is that everyone has the potential to receive answers from within.

SCIENTISTS WHO DISCOVERED SOLUTIONS FROM THEIR DREAMS;

Fredrich August Kekule, a prominent German organic chemist, dreamt of the structure of Benzene. He said, "I sat down writing on my textbook, but the work did not progress. My thought was elsewhere. I turned my chair to the fire and dozed. Again, the atoms were gamboling before my eyes." That was how he discovered the structure of Benzene.

Elias Howe is credited with inventing the sewing machine. "He almost beggared himself before he discovered where the eye of the sewing machine's needle should be located... he might have failed altogether if he had not dreamed he was building a sewing machine for a savage king in a strange country. Just as in his actual working experience, he was perplexed about the needle's eye. He thought the king gave him twenty-four hours to complete the machine and make it sew. If not concluded within the stipulated time, death would be the punishment. Howe worked and worked, puzzled, and finally gave it up. Then he thought he was taken out to be executed, and he noticed that the warriors carried spears pierced near the head. Instantly came the solution to the difficulty, and while the inventor was begging for time, he awoke.

It was 4 am. He jumped out of bed, ran to his workshop, and by 9 am, a needle with an eye at the point had been rudely modeled. After that, it was easy. That is the true story of an essential incident in the invention of sewing machine." [The Bemis History and Genealogy].

Paul McCartney; Music that inspires music

In 1965, Paul McCartney composed the entire melody for the hit acoustic song "Yesterday" in a dream. It came back to him fully formed when he woke up, and he quickly replicated the song on his piano. He asked his friends and family if they'd ever heard it before. He was initially worried that he was simply replicating someone else's work (known as cryptomnesia).

For a month, he went round to people in the music business and asked them whether they had heard it before. Eventually, it became like handing something to the police. If no one claimed it after a few weeks, I could have it.

Lennon and McCartney then wrote lyrics to the melody, and the song was credited to Lennon-McCartney on their album Help!

However, as a melancholy acoustic song involving a solo performance from McCartney and none of the other Beatles, the band members vetoed the release as a UK single that year. It was released in America. "Yesterday" stayed at number one on the Billboard Hot 100 chart for four weeks. It remains massively popular today with more than 2,200 cover versions by other artists, including Aretha Franklin, Katy Perry, The Mamas, and the Papas,

Michael Bolton, Bob Dylan, Ray Charles, and Elvis Presley, Billy Dean, and others. [World of lucid dreaming by Rebecca Turner]

Frederick Banting: Advances in Medicine.

''After his mother passed from diabetes, Frederick Banting was motivated to find a cure. Eventually, he found the next best thing: a treatment using insulin injections that, though not an actual cure, could at least significantly extend the lifespan of sufferers. The discovery won him a Nobel Prize in Medicine at 32 years old. Although he lacked knowledge of diabetes and clinical research. His unique knowledge of surgery and his assistant's (Charles Best's) knowledge of diabetes made the ideal research team. While seeking to isolate the exact cause of diabetes, Banting had a dream telling him to surgically ligate (tie up) the pancreas of a diabetic dog to stop the flow of nourishment. He did and discovered a disproportionate balance between sugar and insulin.'' World of Lucid Dreaming by Rebecca Turner]

Many more solutions have been discovered through dreams.

Train yourself to listen to your internal GPS; learn to trust your instinct. It's God shooting solutions to your mind and giving you directions.

But the method of receiving is different:
Some in pictures while conscious [vision]
Some in pictures while unconscious [dream]
Some hear clearly from within

A quiet mind is vital for receiving. It takes a quiet mind to receive. Albert got one of his equations [E=mc^2 speed of light] from his dream. How? Where did the knowledge come from inside of him? What's inside of him produces that solution? He didn't hear a loud voice. So, what's inside of him produces that solution? What exactly is giving out this information? What's that thing that provides the information internally? What's that thing that speaks to you, and you see what you've heard come to pass? What exactly is it? Medically there is no name for it, and it can't be seen physically.

If something within can provide a solution for you and gives you the correct information about yourself, then it has to be a genius, guardian, and all-knowing. I call the genius on the inside of you the Internal GPS. When you have a challenge, the internal GPS is there to help you out, all you have to do is tune in.

Internal GPS:

Every product works the way the manufacturer has programmed them. So, there is an element of the manufacturer in every product he makes. Same as you, there is an element of God in you that directs and propel you towards destiny. I call it the internal GPS. For instance, software is programmed to guide how the phone works. If a virus comes in, it will affect the programming, and the phone will start to malfunction.

Have you ever heard a voice tell you this is going to happen, and it did happen? You often don't believe it because there is no evidence to back it up.

OR

Have you ever felt there is something wrong about a thing even though looking at it, nothing seems wrong; but you feel from within, something is wrong, later you find what was wrong and you were like, I said it that something isn't right about this thing, that's the internal GPS directing you. The internal GPS communicates in various ways; some see in pictures while some hear... It, therefore, behooves you to be able to discover its operational mode in you, beginning with the ability to look inward. At the same time, you give yourself attention and listen to yourself while you must become conscious of a particular source of information inside of you that is true and perfect.

If you are not conscious of the internal GPS, it will seem non-existent. It doesn't talk every time. Most times, it's heard when the mind is quiet, and some are too scared to listen. The Internal GPS constantly communicates to you who you are meant to be from childhood. It also shares your dreams with you. Sometimes, the dreams are too big for the mind to comprehend. The internal GPS constantly reminds you who you are meant to be. It shows you pictures. When life challenges have suppressed a man's dream, the internal GPS tries to remind you of every available opportunity for resuscitation. It does not leave you completely vulnerable. This is why you're responsible for your rising or down sitting. Being aligned with the internal GPS saves you of unnecessary problems, making you a conduit of solutions to your challenges and a source of inspiration, revelation, and solutions to people and society. Always listen to the internal GPS.

Have you ever thought about why people meditate, fast, pray and do yoga? They want to be connected to their internal GPS. You'll hear people say, "Listen to yourself' all the answers you'll ever need lie within." They are talking about the internal GPS. Your future is inside you, not ahead of you. If you want to know your future, listen the internal GPS.

I didn't hear a loud voice to tell me about my destiny and purpose; I received most of them in the place of prayers. The mind doesn't understand heaven's language [tongues], so as I pray in tongues, the mind is quiet, and the voice of the internal GPS becomes very loud and clear. Sometimes, I don't even prepare to hear, but the moment I start praying, I start hearing. Some days, I just lay on my bed after long hours of studying, and immediately I lay on my bed, I start hearing from the internal GPS. The internal GPS doesn't know if you are a Christian, Muslim, or Buddhist; you have access as long as you are Gods creation.

The primary purpose of religion is to teach you how to have a relationship with your maker through internal GPS. Ignorance about the internal GPS doesn't deny its existence.

From childhood, I would hear a voice speak to me, tell me things that would happen, and when they eventually happened. I would say to myself or anyone around me, I knew that was going to happen, or I heard that such was going to happen. Hence, I could feel an impression that such was going to happen. I have experienced that many times but never believed the voice and so can't differentiate it from my mind speaking as what the voice tells me. It happens repeatedly, so I began to trust it. But I still do not take it seriously.

I remember a day in my primary school I was in stage 6. This faithful evening, as I jumped on my bed, which was the upper bunk, I heard the calm, smooth voice again, saying, "Switch off your phone because, from tomorrow, the boarding students will not be allowed to use mobile phones" It just didn't make sense to me. As I got to the assembly ground, I was a bit late. The first thing I heard them talk about was that the boarding students wouldn't be allowed to use mobile phones anymore. I was amazed, and again, I said, "I heard this yesterday night!"

Something told me they would stop us from using mobile phones. I called the internal GPS "Something" for a long time. As I grow older, I hear people talk about "Tiny Little Voice" or "Still Small Voice."

I asked, "How do I recognize the tiny little voice?"

What does the tiny little voice talk about?

At a point, I stop to fret about the tiny little voice and live my life.

PASSION

"Life is a school where you learn how to remember what your soul already knows." Anonymous

In my primary school years, I love debate. I was always excited when the opportunity for debates came up. Though I was always excited, at the same time, I could be scared, pondering if I was good enough. I was shy, but I was passionate about speaking. The debate was where a part of me could find expression. when the course for debate arise, I feel happy and leap for joy, but my fear and doubts about my competence cause me to retreat. In my Senior Secondary School years, I noticed how passionate I was about speaking and writing, particularly in educational activities. I always love to inform people, educate, sensitize, and proffer solutions to any entangled course. I was a science student, so it was expected of me to be in math or jet club in my school; guess what, I joined press club and was so happy about it. "Now, I can read the news some Fridays," I said. Later, I'll become the editor-in-chief of the press club. Now! I read news for my school most Fridays. Thus, compiling news information wasn't easy, but the joy to read the news fuelled my desire to compile the news.

In primary school, I noticed my passion for speaking found expression during a debate. In secondary school, I noticed my passion for writing and speaking found expressed in the press club. If I wasn't exposed to debate and press club, the writing and speaking part of me might not have found an expression that early. Yet, they were somewhere within me.

What was your passion in primary and secondary school? You might have left primary school many years ago. But, take some minutes to remember what you love doing in your primary and secondary school. The things you liked but were shy to do or didn't feel you had enough confidence to do them.

Primary School:

....

....

....

Secondary School:

....

....

....

Both debate and press club required me to write and speak. The link is writing and speaking at both primary and secondary schools. What's the link between what excites you in primary and secondary school?

....

....

....

IMPROVEMENT

"Do it again. Play it again. Sing it again. Reread it. Write it again. Sketch it again. Rehearse it again. Rerun it. Try it again.

Because again is practice, and practice is an improvement, and improvement only leads to perfection."　　　— *Richelle E. Goodrich.*

Though, I love writing. Yet, every time I write, I always feel, I need to Improve. My first three semesters in senior secondary school exposed me to writing. In that class, you have to learn a lot about essay writing. I was always excited to write. But, whenever I was done, I would feel, "I need to do better" This feeling held me back from continuous writing or giving my writing to people to read. I started reading educative books in year one of Senior Secondary School, so it provoked the writing part of me. Looking back, I would have gotten a teacher to help improve my writing. But today, I can decide to use editors, learn online [courses, you tube], or any English corrector apps like Grammarly.

My gifts were my hobbies for a long time. People would visit me, and before I knew it, I had a serious conversation with them. Every part of them was listening, and from their countenance, I could tell there was total concentration or rapt attention to the conversation. The look on their faces, sitting position, gestures, and atmosphere indicated absolute concentration. Sometimes, it might be unpremeditated, but I noticed most of my conversations go in that line. I don't want to sound like a teacher to a friend I should be chatting with. I sometimes don't even know where those words are coming from. When I'm done speaking, I will regurgitate any new word I said for the first time while listening to myself again because I was hearing it for the first time. It became what excites me, people would come to me for advice, and I would effortlessly pour myself into them.

The words I just said to this person are not mine; where did they come from? I would ask myself. One day, I was scared I would lose the wisdom I had, and I might not be able to advise people again. But immediately, I heard from the Internal GPS say "Don't worry, you won't lose it." I just started reading educative books for more knowledge. The truth is, the wisdom was not from the books I read. It was deeper. It came from the manifestation of the Holy Spirit in me. The Spirit of God is the spirit of revelation and inspiration.

In my early university days, I realized that speaking was a gift for me. I would find myself speaking to people for hours, trying to educate them in one area of life or the other. I wouldn't mind spending hours without food for as long as I was impacting lives, changing people's perceptions, and investing positively into people's lives. Each word has a way of hitting me while changing and correcting one side of me and the other. Also, I realized there was massive strength with which I attend to two or three different people at a stretch, spending a minimum of 1hour or more with each person. I was always excited about doing this. I do it effortlessly.

As I began to listen to messages and read more educative books, there was massive improvements and transformation within a few months. Indeed, it goes beyond the educative books I was reading. I would say things have never read about. So, I realized it was

God's wisdom at work in me. Don't stop at making your gift a hobby, ensure you refine them by learning to become excellent at them. Endeavor to get materials and people that can help you improve or become better at the gift.

What are your gift?

....

....

....

What are your plans to improve or become better at your gift?

....

....

....

Who is doing great at your gift that you can learn from? Mention 3 names:

....

....

....

How can you connect with their materials? YouTube, DVD, Podcasts, Online courses, Conferences, Seminars

....

....

....

At some point in life, people will voice out your gift.

You'll hear them make a statement like this, "Oh! You are good at this; I think you should take it more seriously. Or, "Oh! I came to you because I knew you are good at it". Sometimes, you reply might be, "Oh! I just like doing it" those things you like doing and do effortlessly are your gifts. When you hear words like that, take note.

YOU TEACH BETTER THAN US:

I was preparing for the West African Senior School Certificate Examination final exam in my final year in Secondary School. My friends and I decided we'll leave the hostel every night to study. We shared the topic of a subject among ourselves. Each person had a topic to teach others. I was the first to teach the first night I taught them, and they understood based on the positive reactions that ensued. Then, as the next person came up to teach, I had to stop her at some point. I didn't understand what she was teaching, and I voiced out. She explained again, but that did not make any difference. I resolved within myself "I would go and read this again." At the end of the study, I repeated, I didn't understand what you were teaching, and one of them replied "Betty! We are not like you, don't expect us to teach like you. " I replied her being peeved when she said it many years back, it didn't make sense to me. Looking back now I realized she simply voiced out my gift.

A person can have a teaching profession but might not be a teacher. Teaching is a gift. Training and technicalities are required for effective teaching. Though, it can be earned as a skill. But it's a gift some were born with and should still be refined. If not refined, someone that learned the skills might become better. Every element of gifts in you leaves you with the assignment of self-improvement and validation. Development of your gift is essential. Remember, as beautiful as a pen is, it needs to be sharpened before use, so are your gifts. There are processes to its operation, channeling, harnessing, and propagation. Hence, you have to be intentional about the content, how to use it and where it can function most. This is what makes your gift of high value and profit to God, you, and society. You must refine your gifts.

YOUR WORDS ARE POWERFUL.

I went to a friend's birthday party and was told I would speak. I simply asked myself what am I going to say, I said I would freestyle, but I knew if I opened my mouth, I would voice out words of wisdom (It is just who I am, it's my gift that has been refined and yet remains at the drilling stage). Before I knew it, I was handed the microphone, and I started speaking, I got the audience's attention, and the room went quiet that a drop of water would make a difference. At some point, I could feel goose bumps as I was speaking out wisdom and couldn't control it. When I was done speaking, the first thing I said to myself was, those are not my words. But, this time I know where they came from. Immediately after the party, my friend walked up to me and said," Hey Betty, those words you spoke were inspiring and powerful. You are very good at speaking". She said much more, saying, "You have to take it seriously. It wasn't the first time the Internal GPS spoke through me, so I wasn't surprised.

PAY THE PRICE TO GET BETTER AT YOUR GIFT.

Everything you want in life is achievable but has a price. Nothing is easy or free. If you don't pay the price for success, you'll inadvertently pay the price for failure. It's your choice to pick the type of price you want to pay. Emotions are like pointers showing us what we need to pay attention to. If you don't feel confident about your gift, work on yourself. Your confidence matters in expressing your gift. Express your gifts flawlessly, confidence is quite important. In a situation whereby you have come on the average, you can be sure of perfection when the little you have is attached with confidence which is the "I Can" spirit.

No one is born with confidence. The things we do is what brings confidence. You'll simply gain confidence as you learn and practice your gift repeatedly. Repetition is said to be the mother of all skills.

NO PRICE IS TOO HIGH TO GET BETTER AT YOUR GIFT.

If you want to succeed with your gift, it's necessary to develop it. You see people's success and not necessarily their level of hard work. People are rewarded publicly for what they practice privately It's not going to be easy, but I promise you, it is worth it. The time, effort & resources at the end of the day are always worth it. Be determined to improve your gifts and not stop having them as hobby. The different between good and great is the willingness to sacrifice.

Pay the price to improve your gift, and keep improving your gift. The more you improve your gift, the more valuable you become. People pay for values. People far and near would pay thousands of dollars to watch Michael Jackson sing and dance live, so why will they do that? Anyone in their neighborhood could sing and dance better than Michael Jackson. But, the person in the neighborhood hasn't developed the required value and network, so he's not as valuable as Michael Jackson, who had worked immensely to improve his gift. Refine your gift to become valuable. Your value will determine how much you'll make in life.

Are you willing to pay the price to make your gift valuable?

....

If yes, what price are you willing to pay?

....

....

....

If you don't have money, are you willing to start saving to get the necessary teachings and materials? Remember, people pay for values.

....

....

....

EXISTING BUT NOT LIVING.

You can be alive and not living.

Existing is when you allow life to happen to you; you accept life.

Living is when you happen to life. You lead life. Living requires effort, unlike existing.

Living is when you are intentional about your life.

The World Health Organization (WHO) defines an adolescent as anyone between ages 10 and 19. Adolescence is a transitional phase of growth and development between childhood and adulthood. Centers for Diseases Control and Prevention [CDCP] went further to group the adolescence age into stages:

9-11 –Middle Childhood

12-14 – Young Teenagers

15-17 - Teenagers

Each phase has its developmental milestones. For instance, age 9-11years is when a child grows independent from family and interest in friend become apparent. Ages12-14years is a time of physical, mental, emotional, and social changes. Hormones change as puberty begins. 15-17years is a time of changes for how teenagers think, feel, and interact with others and how their bodies develop.

At age16, I got into medical school. Psychologically at this age, I was expected to have a change of thought, feelings, and interactions with others. I was expected to gradually transition into the adulthood stage.

As a 100-level medical student, part of the curriculum was to take some significant introductory science courses like Mathematics, Physics, Biology, and Chemistry. We had mathematics almost every day and a lot of impromptu tests. At least one lecturer would say to the class each day, "Not all of you will be promoted to the 200 level. Some of you will be move to another department. Every time I hear this word, I always say in my mind, "I don't want to disappoint my parent." It was an expensive school, one of the best in Nigeria. I hear these words almost daily. My fear grew and was constantly triggered.

It was 100 level. I was meant to socialize but couldn't. I was mentally blocked and tried to pass 100level to 200 level. Socialization was not in my vocabulary. My fear grew daily. I didn't want to disappoint my parents. They've spent so much on me. I grew up in a polygamous extended family. My culture presumes that when a child fails, it's a shame to the parents, especially the mother. I didn't want that to happen.

Many days, I would pick my book, read and stare at it but not study. I was so afraid that my brain couldn't remember what I read most of the time. Close to examination week, I would jump up from the bed like I was being chased to study. I was lost mentally, emotionally, spiritually, and even physically. Despite all these, peer influence was trying to find expression. I remember going to class one day, and I began to feel, "I didn't dress well," and my clothes didn't look good. Just that moment, I heard what my mum always says to me, "Betty! You're beautiful, and there is nothing you wear that doesn't look good on you. That was what saved me that day. I might have gone back to the hostel to change or ignore going to class, and on many other days, my mummy's voice kept returning to my head. Her voice invariably helped me overcome the peer group influence".

SURVIVAL MODE.

I was just existing! Food and movies were my coping mechanisms. Thank God my dad sends sufficient money monthly. I had enough money to eat. When I'm not so happy, I will go to the cafeteria and buy rice as usual (the typical food) with chicken and juice to allay my fears and difficulties. Surprisingly, my fear grew that if someone came into my room and shut the door, I could feel the sound in my heart, and it felt like my heart was heavy or would just drop off. No doubt, I was drenched with fear. When the fear became overwhelming, I would find my way home. Going home was therapeutic for me. It was as if no one was seeing the real struggle I was going through. Physically, I became emaciated, all my younger siblings were chubby or robust. My dad would always remark, "Don't you eat? I knew within me, I fed well.

While all these were going on, I heard some people remark, "She is not friendly, she doesn't play with people, and she doesn't talk to people. How can I? My internal conversation was more than the external. I was losing myself daily. Nothing practically excites me.

Fear was eating me up, and I didn't like that. I was scared of everything at that moment but adapted to it. I didn't know that intense fear wasn't normal. So, I was never taught something was wrong with me. If I was asked, I might not be able to explain what was happening to me at that point in my life. The truth is, I was in the process of re-setting my mind, trying to change my mode of thinking, feelings, and interactions with others. I wasn't aware of this, so all I did was keep to myself because I didn't understand what was happening. How do I explain to others what I don't understand myself? I was just existing!

FALL BACK ON RELIGION.

I grew up in the typical African Christian home. If you have a problem, the next thing is to run to God, and they do not tell you this most times. You see the elders do it and you take in the mentality. As my fear grew, my heart felt like it was going to drop when I heard a loud sound. I said to myself that the only way to pass and scale through 100 to 2001 is God. I joined the prayer department. Many nights I would jump up to pray or dance to God. I would pray and go back to my bed to sleep when I was done. It was a one-way conversation. I don't hear God speak after one hour of conversation with Him, not that God doesn't speak, but I have not trained myself to hear from Him.

I was just religious and had no relationship with God. Yes, I was in the prayer department. I prayed for at least one hour each day, but there was no relationship with God. I was a churchgoer, and I didn't miss Sunday services. I love God and would be in any gathering held to honor Him. But I was not in a relationship with Him. So, my conversation is mostly one way, and that was me talking to God. I was praying, yet, growing in fear every day.

MEET THE INTERNAL GPS.

GPS is a positioning system based on a satellite network continuously transmits coded information. The information transmitted from the satellites can be interpreted by receivers to precisely identify locations on earth by measuring distances from the satellites.

THREE COMPONENTS OF GPS

Space segment: The satellites orbiting the earth transmit timing and ranging messages.

Control Segment: This monitors the health and position of the satellites in the space segment and transmits correct information back up to the satellites.

User segment: The handheld or other receivers interpret the satellite's messages.

Mechanism of the GPS: Information is received from the space segment by the control segment. The control segment also sends information back to the space segment. The control segment receives and sends information to the space segment.

You can see the control segment as God, the space segment as the internal GPS, and the user segment as you. God discusses with the internal GPS, and the internal GPS, in turn, communicates with you. That internal GPS is called the Spirit of God. God is not here on earth, but His Spirit is here. There are many spirits, and you also are one. Demons are spirits too. So, the Spirit of God can also be called Holy Spirit since the Bible clarifies that God is a Spirit and He's holy. Hence, the name Holy Spirit.

RELATIONSHIP WITH INTERNAL GPS

I noticed fellowship was ongoing in the room next to mine for the past few days, and my host's friend came to invite me. As a lover of God, I said okay. That was how I began to attend the fellowship every evening. This was an extension period for medical students. The extension is a moment when the university is on vacation, but medical students are asked to wait behind for extra curriculum activities. In the fellowship, we pray and listen to sermons daily. The first thing I noticed in the fellowship was the act of speaking in tongues. Praying in the spirit was allowed and encouraged, but I don't speak in tongues. One day, my friend, now a sister, walked up to me and said, do you know it's a necessity for every believer to speak in tongues? I replied, "I don't." We don't speak in tongues in my church back home. Moreover, I taught speaking in tongues was for those high up there in the spirit. Therefore, she showed me many scriptures backing what she said up.

Some of the scriptures include:

"And these signs will follow those who believe. In My name, they will cast out demons. they will speak with new tongues, they will take up serpents, and if they drink anything deadly it will by no means hurt them. They will lay hands on the sick, and they will recover……..." Mark 16:15-20.

The scripture above didn't say only pastors, prophets, apostles, or leaders of the church are entitled to the gift. It is simple for anyone who believes In God, in His only begotten Son – Jesus Christ, and has submitted his or her life unto Him as their Lord and Savior. Hence, the moment you give your life to Jesus, you belong to God. So you have the promise of the Holy Spirit, which is the Spirit of God the Father. One of the pieces of evidence of the presence and the manifestation of the Holy Spirit in you is the ability to speak in tongues.

"For he who speaks in a tongue does not speak to men but God, for no one, understands him; however, in the spirit, he speaks mysteries. Verse 4 says, "He that speaketh in an unknown tongue edifieth himself" 1 Corinthians14:2

She further explained,

When you pray in tongues, you're talking to God and no one. So, people don't have to understand you. God understands what you're saying. When you pray in tongues, you rise like a tower, you are charged up in your inner man.

"And they were all filled with the Holy Ghost, and began to speak with other tongues, as the Spirit gave them utterance." – Acts 2:4 KJV. When you receive the gift of the Holy Spirit, it gives you utterance to speak in tongues. I nodded in unity; I appreciated her and left for my room.

On getting to my room, I knelt beside my bed and asked for the gift of the Holy Spirit and utterance to speak in tongues, and I wasn't done asking. I started saying words I didn't understand. I stopped and said, "Those words can't be from me" I looked around my room. My roommate was not around, and no noisy sound from the environment. Does that mean I just spoke in tongues? That was unbelievable; it can't be this easy, I told myself. While still on my knees, I rest my hand on my bed to continue praying in my understanding. The same word came out. I stopped and said, "Does that mean I have started praying in tongues?'' I still couldn't believe it, so I was shy to tell anyone.

The next day was on Sunday; I went to church, and the pastor said, if you don't speak in tongues, raise your hand. I raised my hand. Before the hand was fully up, I heard clearly and loud enough that I couldn't deny it. "Betty! Stop deceiving yourself; you've started praying in tongues". It was the first time I heard the Holy Spirit clearly and knew it was the Holy Spirit. Remember, I said we listened to some messages every night. The first message I listened to was titled "Who is the Spirit?" By Rev. Chris Oyakilohme. The message explained the role of the Holy Spirit as seen in 1 John 14:16 (AMP version).

And I will ask the Father, and He will give you another] Helper (Comforter, Advocate, Intercessor—Counselor, Strengthener, Standby), to be with you forever —

I had many of Pastor Chris' messages on my gadget. I watched him daily. I began to understand my identity in Christ at 18 years. I started building my relationship with the Holy Spirit; I would pray in tongues daily for minutes or hours, not asking for anything, just to fellowship with God. My life was changing positively, and my fear was leaving gradually without saying goodbye. Fasting was becoming attractive, and I started studying the word of God and trusting the Holy Spirit for revelations. I grew from just studying the book of Psalms and Proverbs.

As I grew in my relationship with the Holy Spirit, my excitement was hearing the Holy Spirit speak to me most during prayers. I would ask Him a lot of questions and listen to Him respond. He would tell me a lot about me; who I was, why I was born. I gradually gained clarity about myself. The response I don't get immediately comes later. I was no longer praying for wisdom because I had begun to spend so much time with wisdom [God], I walked in wisdom, and everyone around me called my attention to it. I remember going to a book shop to get an educative book, the young man I met there listened to me and asked, "What church do you attend?" I said, "Christ Embassy. "He responded, "No wonder your pastor is a man of wisdom.

When I got home, my mindset was that I was done with my parent's church. I heard them call the Holy Spirit in almost everything we do, but they never introduced him to me. How could they do that? So, I made up my mind to greet them bye. They all knew at home that something had changed about this girl. All of them started calling me a Christian. Even though I didn't announce my relationship with the Holy Spirit to them, His presence and manifestation had become evident in me.

One Sunday, I found myself in my parent's church, and I decided I was not going to the adult church but would go to the children's church. I saw a man called Prophet Abiodun Sule teaching the children while he allowed everyone to speak. So, I commented. Later, he walked up to me and asked, "What church do you attend?" I told him, and he said I knew already. I was a cell leader at Christ Embassy in Ukraine, he said. Since then, he has given me materials aligned with destiny and spoken to me and to me.

The person who mentor you during your spiritual development matters. Mentorship is the transfer of mindset. If this is not achieved, you have not been mentored. The goal of mentorship is for the mentor to transfer his mindset to his mentee. I have watched Pastor Chris so much that his mind has been transferred to me. I wasn't conscious of this, but people around me couldn't keep quiet or stop staring at the wonders I had become.

I have always known I love writing and speaking, but as I pray in tongues, it becomes more precise, which also became a searchlight to other potentials within me. As the Spirit of God was teaching me about purpose, I found some messages about Purpose by Dr.

Myles Munroe. Feeding my spirit man daily [praying and listening to sermons] was what gave me joy. I did it passionately. One day, someone slammed the door where I was, and it didn't feel like my heart would drop or be heavy. I was surprised fear had gone. It disappears without bidden me bye. I have listened to many messages about God's love and grace from Joseph Prince and Pastor Chris. I understood His love. I grew in confidence with time.

I got a journal to write down the things Holy Spirit shared with me daily. Holy Spirit became so real than the air I breathe. My life drastically became transformed for good. Being grateful is an understatement. I went from existing to **LIVING!**

It's like the missing part of me was found entirely and coupled back into my system. I simply became revitalized; joy that had been missing for a while came back fully. I became stable. I was giving less attention to my academics, it was stressful for me before, but now, I found one thing I love to do. I didn't know there was a part of me that could still light up the way it did. Every day, I would hear a lot about myself. I would ask my internal GPS questions daily, and this became a source of revolution in my life.

My relationship with the Holy Spirit allays my fear; it was all I needed for spiritual stamina, mental bliss, and better understanding. I watch my life transformed.

The age of 13- 18 is significant, and adolescents try to figure out who they are. Questions of Identity keep running over their minds. They try to fill the void within. Today, a word like "I'm bored" is used. They try to fill the void with relationships, drugs, alcohol, sex, and many other things. Some will date different partners to fill the void, they keep looking for a perfect partner, but they do not realize it's not about the partner but about them. After some might have taken drugs or smoked cigarettes to cushion their boredom, a few minutes or hours after the drugs have been waived off, they are back to reality. This is a fact to show that all these do not solve the problem because if it does, there shouldn't be a relapse.

Terry Perry said, there will always be challenges in life, so parents must teach their children to turn to God. If not, they will turn to something else like drugs, alcohol.

CHAPTER 3

BECOME A DIFFERENT PERSON

"Every next level of your life will demand a different version of you."

If you're going to become successful, you have to understand what stops people from succeeding. Success comes with a price, and you have to be willing to pay the price. The moment you think a price is too high to pay, you have immediately lost in that area. The higher the success, the higher the price. If you are not determined to pay the price for success, don't waste energy desiring it. The journey is not an easy one. It's not a smooth road but a bumpy and rigorous one. Stop wishing success was easier. Your wish won't change the principles and law here on earth. You must brace up and make yourself available to pay the necessary price. No one gets to the top by proxy. It is a combination of many acts and processes. So you must understand that it's not going to be a stroll in the park. Nevertheless, it is quite achievable as long as you believe in yourself and as much as you are determined to be at the top of your game. At the same time, you possess discipline, diligence, courage, determination, faith, focus, foresight, self-control, and others.

Success is predictable.

God designs life to function by principles. Rain falls on the good and the bad. Don't wish situations are better and wish you were better to handle the situation. The principles will not change for you. God doesn't even go against these principles except in rare circumstances. Regardless of your race, religion, tribe, culture, and environment, the principles are the same if you implement them, you will automatically get the right result. You simply have the result of whatever you have done, so a wrong motive cannot produce a right action. In all sincerity, God has designed the world in a way that what you do is what will determine your advancement or greatness in life. This has nothing to do with religion, race, ethnicity, and the rest. That is why a diligent handicap can get the best out of life than a lazy sane mind and perfect body. On the other hand, a lazy man cannot have the same measure of blessing as the diligent. So, you'll embrace ashes when you have done nothing with your life.

The dream of greatness for a lazy man is like a hungry man opening his mouth into the air, some principles guide every life affair. So, it behooves you to look inward to know what you need to do per time and regarding those aspects of your life where you're experiencing downturns or debacles. The ability to do the right thing within the circle will automatically bring great rewards for you in time.

People are rewarded publicly for what they practice privately. Most people overestimate what they can do in a year and underestimate what they can do in a decade – Tony Robbins.

To become successful, you have to be ready for success. Pay the price, and play full out. Success doesn't come to those that dabble; (one leg in, one leg out). Success doesn't come to those that are not sure they will be successful. Most successful people will tell you, I know I was going to succeed. The conviction gets them going when it's tough on the journey to success. Ask yourself, "Are you ready for success?" No doubt, it's not an easy road, but I promise you it is worth it. On the journey of success, transition is inevitable, while in transition, you have to surrender to become a different version of yourself.

Frustration:

When it's time to become a different version of you, frustration is the first sign that shows often. You'll become uncomfortable about how things are, you might be complaining before, but this time, it has grown intensively. Everything around you seem to piss you off. Every area of your life seems to be breaking down, and it's like everything and everyone is getting on your nerves simultaneously. Your value and standard need an upgrade because it's no longer working for you. You know practically something is wrong but can't exactly pinpoint what it is. You're in a surviving mood. You try to figure out what you're not doing right. When you feel this way, it's a sign that indicates a move to the next level of your life. Frustration shows up because you can't step to the next level with the old version of you.

At this point, two things happen. Either you go back to your comfort zone and continue living the old version of yourself, or you become a different version of yourself and step to the next level of your life. Many don't know they are in transition, so they fight to return to their comfort zones, and you hear words like, "This is the way I do it" nothing is wrong with that. But the question is, how should you do it now? You did it that way before, but it's no longer working. You should ask how I can make it work. To answer this question requires mental work. It requires thinking. Many don't like the word "thinking," so they run away from it and stay in their comfort zones. The brain also doesn't like to use energy to learn new things. So, it supports you to remain in your comfort zone - the familiar zone. If you want to attain a new level, you have to be inconvenient till the time the new possibility is birthed.

In the middle stage of transition

You will observe many lonely times; I mean isolation. This time allows you to reflect on yourself and the possibilities ahead. It allows you to listen to yourself. You speak to yourself more and what you have to say; this period allows the internal GPS voice to be louder than ever. Just like the internal GPS does, it will guide and direct you if you acknowledge the GPS can. You want to eliminate as many people as possible at this stage. Sometimes, you can intentionally cut some people off because you think you are losing focus because of them, but that's not true. It's time to listen to destiny on the next assignment you have to deliver. Until you cooperate with destiny, it will continue to frustrate you, till you become uncomfortable with the old level and version of you.

The last phase of transition

You know you're coming out of transition if you surrender to become a different version of yourself. When you embrace the uncertainty, when you agree to learn, unlearn, and relearn when you say words like;

"I don't know what this will be like, but I'm trying it."
"I'm just going to behold a new version of me."
"I'm tired of where I am; I need to move forward."
"I'm just going to trust God!!
"I know there is more inside of me; I'm going to unleash it, I might not know how, but I will find how."

At this stage, you know you have to become a different person. You can no longer continue to think or behave the way you used too. You have to leave your limiting beliefs behind, and be clear about what you're transiting into. The struggle of returning to the old version of you will spring up but remind yourself how the new version of you behave, or you say, the new me has to behave differently to achieve the following vision God wants me to execute. You have to permit yourself to be clothed with the new mindset, behavior, and action of the new version of you. You have to be patient with yourself as your creator reviews a part of you that you don't even know. Be patient with your creator as He unravels the mystery you are.

You can't predict the transition time frame, but you must surrender yourself to learn, unlearn & relearn; this will play a significant role in you coming out of transition quickly. It could last for months or years if you don't know you are in transition. You might not be conscious of learning, unlearn and relearn.

Do you think you are in transition?
If yes, continue with the questions below:
If not, you can continue reading:
Don't hold back any words from your mind; write them all out. I mean, write exclusively, and pour out your thoughts.

What phase of transition are you

Early

Middle

Late

What signs made you pick your answer?

....

....

....

Are you willing to surrender to meet a new version of yourself?

....

If not, what's stopping you? I mean, what's your excuse?

....

....

....

Are the above mentioned things stopping you, or are you permitting them?

....

....

....

Think deeper, are the lists above really stopping you, or you're speaking from a place of fear?

....

....

....

One more time, are they stopping you, or you're scared you don't know what it will cost you.

....

....

....

If everything works out fine, will you be willing to surrender?

....

....

....

Have faith that it will work out fine.
You can't see it but trust your creator. He's more committed to your success than ever imagined.

What are you willing to do to become a new version of yourself?

....

....

....

What belief are you willing to let go of to become a new version of yourself?

....

....

....

What belief are you taking to become the version needed for the next level?

....
....
....

What behaviors do you have to leave behind?

....
....
....

What behaviors do you have to take on to become a new version of yourself?

....
....
....

What actions are you willing to take to become a different version of yourself?

....
....
....

DECISION

It is in your moment of decision that your destiny is shaped. – Tony Robbins.

The first step to change is exposure. If you're not exposed to something different, you won't question the present belief. If you don't question your present belief, you can't change the belief. If you don't change your belief, you can't change your behavior. Your behavior determine your destiny.

A decision can be good but not right; to make the right decision, you need the right information; to have the right information, you have to be intentional about it. To be intentional, you need to be genuine and willing to change. The quality of information you have will shape your belief system, and your belief system will determine the quality of your decisions. To make the right decision, you need the right mindset.

I want to invest in crypto currency.

That's a good decision.

So, I will pick any coin and buy then leave it for some years.

That's not the right decision.

Why?

Because leaving a coin for many years doesn't guarantee it will pump up, so many coins have not been pumped in years.

The right information is vital for the right belief system. If you want the right information about something, go to those doing the same thing you want with proven results. I mean, learn from those in the field with proven results; they have books, videos on YouTube, seminars, conferences, and probably a course today. Immerse yourself into their materials till you're sure you have the right information you need to execute; they are called mentors or coaches; you can also reach out to them to mentor/ coach you personally if need be.

Mentors are those who have walked in your shoes, passed through it, and have the experience. They can tell you how to get results faster when they mentor you. What took your mentor ten years can take you a few weeks or months? Mentors share information that helps you go faster and stronger. Trying to figure out things yourself is the old way of doing things. You might get the result you want after many months or years. To prevent doing things that won't get you the result you want, pay a mentor for speed; they'll tell you what to do and what not to do. They'll help you get unstuck when you get stuck because they have been there.

Mentorship is the transfer of the mentor's mindset to the mentee; you know you have been genuinely mentored by a person when you start thinking like them. Until the mind is changed; you can't get a new result. When you gain the mindset of your mentor, getting the same result as your mentor is only a matter of time.

BELIEF:
"The man who says he can, and the man who says he can't are both correct." -Confucius

Before you make a decision, check if you have a limiting belief; limiting belief sounds like excuse. I should have started that business, but my family members were not supportive.

I can't survive without him/her.
All online businesses are scams.
All males are scum.

There is no true love.
This Christianity thing is not working;
I don't have enough money to save.
I can't do it.
A single parent raised me, which is why I'm like this.
If my mummy were better than she was, I would be a better person.
If only my parent were rich, I would be rich by now.
If my father were alive, all this wouldn't be happening to me.
I'm too old, and I can't start all over.
If only my husband or wife borrowed me that money.
Where will I start from?
My life is finished.
If God says it, it's going to happen.
My husband is stopping me from living the life I want.

Every time you say or make an excuse like this, question the excuse

e.g.

Is it true that my life is ruined?

Is it true that, if my father is alive, all this won't be happening?

"It is your decisions, not your conditions that determine your destiny." – Tony Robbins.

What will you focus on when there is always something wrong and something right? Where focus goes, energy goes. Limiting belief will prevent you from taking full responsibility for yourself. As long as you blame someone for your situation, you can't experience change, and you need to take full responsibility for your life. Your life is a physical manifestation of the thoughts in your head.

Say it out loud,

My life is the total of every decision I have made and still making. I'm like this because I choose to be, consciously or unconsciously. You hear people say, **"That's the way I am."** That's not how you are but how you choose to be. You were not born that way; your experience has shaped you in that manner. Disempowering your limiting belief so you won't live all your life just existing, surviving daily when you could thrive. I mean, if you'll permit yourself, you will soar.

THE BRAIN MAKES MISTAKE.

It's said that the average adult makes about 35000 decisions a day – newspaper USA today. Have you ever found yourself in a scenario where you try to let someone see from your view because you have the right information? Still, they won't. They believe the wrong information they have is the right one and they argue passionately with the wrong information. You wonder, how in the world can this person think this way? It's because the information they have fed their brain is wrong. They believe with all their might that is the right information. Those wrong ideologies were formed by the wrong information saved in the brain. The brain can only give you back the information you have saved. If you save wrong information, you will misbelieve and in turn, make wrong decisions. When the brain makes mistakes, it never agrees it has made mistakes. It just simply continues to function as if nothing wrong has happened.

The brain will automatically reject the information that it is not conversant with. When you take in information for the first time, and you don't go back again, the brain will consider them not important and delete them. When you have taken in the information over and over. It becomes registered in your subconscious mind, and the brain will consider it important and save it. When you hear a new word or new information, it's not your intellect that hears it first, but your emotions. The brain gives an emotional resistance to new information.

To change the wrong information the brain has saved, you have to denounce the wrong directives. **You get stuck most times because the brain doesn't know what to do next.** You know it's a wrong directive because you're not getting the desired result. The only way to get unstuck is to feed the brain with new information. You must repeat for the brain to consider important to save them. The brain has saved those limiting beliefs, and you need to disempower them to delete them. We can't get rid of a pattern without replacing it with a new one. Relapse will happen. As we disempower limiting beliefs, we have to replace them with empowering beliefs; new exposure triggers change if they cause us to question our beliefs. Whenever we believe something, we no longer question it in any way.

DISEMPOWER LIMITING BELIEF.

The first step to changing a limiting belief is to question it

Ask questions about it

· Where did I get this belief?

· What has it cost me before, and what will it continue to cost me?

Let's do this together:

If you're still wondering what your limiting beliefs are; they sound like excuse.

A. List your goals, your top 3 goals

....

....

....

Goal 1

What excuse have you been giving yourself? List as many as possible.

....

....

....

Goal 2

....

....

....

Goal 3

....
....
....

B. Where/who did I get each limiting belief? Is it worth emulating to achieve this goal?

Goal 1

....
....
....

Goal 2

....
....
....

Goal 3

....
....
....

D. What has this belief cost me?

Financially:

....
....
....

Physically:

....

....

....

Relationships:

....

....

....

 Family/loved ones:

....

....

....

E. What will this belief cost me if I don't change?

 Financially:

....

....

....

Physically:

....

....

....

Relationships:

....

....

....

 Family/loved ones:

....
....
....

F. Write the empowering belief for each goal now to replace the limiting belief. You know the limiting beliefs are lies, write the truth now.

Goal 1

....
....
....

Goal 2

....
....
....

Goal 3

....
....
....

Now that you've answered the questions, you must be committed to informing your brain about the new decision for a minimum of 30 days. Research says that it takes 21days to form new habits and 66 days for a new behavior to become automatic. You can dedicate 10mins a day to looking at empowering and disempowering beliefs.

BELIEF TO HAVE FOR CHANGE TO TAKE PLACE:

Firstly, you must believe there is a problem.

Secondly, you must believe you can solve the problem.

Thirdly, you must believe you have to solve it now.

Fourthly, you must believe you can.

Lastly, maintain the belief to prevent relapse. Relapse occurs if you are unclear about what you want and why you want it.

CLARITY:

When people think they have a time management problem, I believe it is clarity, not time management- Dean Graziosi.

If you are not clear about what you want and why you want it, you will give up your goals easily. If you are not passionate about it, you can't fully commit. To achieve your goals, you need not just the external force but the internal force. This internal force comes from a place of conviction. When no one is clapping, the internal force is what will keep propelling you. When you're clear about what you want, you set your mind. When your mind is prepared, it's easier for your body to carry out the information. That's why it's said to write out your goals a night before; it allows the brain to work on the information overnight. Your actions are almost automatic if you're clear about what you wrote when you get up the following day. If you don't distract yourself, you will have a productive day.

Your body can't go where your mind has never been; to achieve your goal your mind must first see the goal and believe it has happened. The mind doesn't know the past or future. It only knows the present. So, when your mind believes the goal has happened and replays it in your head, achieving them becomes easy. To the mind, it has happened. So, it summons all the inner energy needed to make it happen.

The holy bible tells us. "Faith is the *assurance* of things *hoped* for, the evidence of things not seen [*the conviction of their reality*]. Faith comprehends the fact that physical senses cannot experience. –Hebrew 11:1AMP

Hope is being expectant; assurance means Confirmation of something. So, faith is the Confirmation of what you're expecting, you have not seen it physically, but you expect it so much that your mind creates a picture as if it has happened. You expect it so much, and you feel like it has happened. Until you see it in your mind, you can't have it. If you have it, you will lose it because your mind doesn't understand it and can't manage it.

WHAT DO YOU DO WHEN YOUR MIND SUBMITS TO A VISION OR DISAGREE WITH A VISION?

You have to start taking in new information to support your new idea or vision, start learning about it, watch videos and books related to your new topic, and go to conferences and seminars related to your new subject of study. Also, you might get a mentor in that area to get your mind familiar with the topic. At first, it will be new to your brain, but as you continue to educate your mind about it, the mind will gradually begin to understand. As the mind understands the information, it begins to absorb and agree with your vision and ideas. To be clear about what you want, you have to be intentional. So, when the answer comes, we can recognize it.

QUESTIONS OF CLARIFICATION:

A. What do I want?

B. How can I achieve it; list them out in steps?

C. Why do I want it?

D. What skills and capabilities do I need to achieve it?

DIARY OR JOURNAL.

The main difference between diary and journal is the intention behind the writing. The diary records what's happening daily, while the journal helps reflect on your life, and its purpose varies. It could be for academics, gratitude, goal settings, travel, note, business, dreams, and many more.

DIARY:

"Keep a daily diary of your dreams, goals, and accomplishments. If your life is worth living, it's worth recording."

– Marylyn Grey

Diary is for writing down what happens in our lives daily. I love to pen down what God shares with me. I love to write down my experience each day in my journal. I have been using a diary for over 5years. Every time I go back to read them and note the first day an idea comes to my mind and how it became a reality, the feeling is surreal. It could be the things God said He would do for me, and now it has happened but doesn't even remember He said it. On many occasions, God had referred me back to my diary to confirm some past experiences and promises which have become a reality; they simply help us to track our growth and the date an event happens.

JOURNAL

"Journaling is paying attention to the inside to live well from the inside out." – Lee Wise.

Journaling is writing down our thoughts for the progressive result of ideas. The ability to write down your thoughts exposes you to the conversations in your soul and spirit. As you write, you'll become clear about the purpose of a thing, mysteries of life [including why you are here on planet earth], ideas will spring up, and you'll become more conscious of your dreams, you can trace where your fears and worries stem out from through your writing.

Journaling calms the mind, brings you the consciousness of your thoughts, and helps you know your desires. Also, it helps us to be clear about what we want. It helps us listen to ourselves, and this result in you loving yourself. Journaling is a means of giving attention to yourself; it helps us arrange our thoughts. When this happens, we feel good as a hormone called feeling good is secreted; after that, you'll experience peace. Journal enables you to trace where your emotions stem from, it helps you to focus, it moves you towards your goals, it keeps your brain sharp, it triggers you to be grateful, it helps to reduce stress, depression, and anxiety, and it's said to improve your immune system. It boosts your mood, increases your self-esteem, strengthens your emotional function, boosts your creativity, and helps you sleep better.

As we become conscious of ourselves, our limiting beliefs are exposed, and we can address them. If you ask me which to get [journal or diary], I suggest you get the two.

Step to journal daily:
· Get a journal or an exercise book to write
· Choose a convenient location and place
· Determine how many minutes you want to journal.

Set alarm for the time; until the time is up, don't stand up. I suggest you start with 15mins daily, from there to 30mins and 1 hour. If nothing is coming, ask questions.

Use clarity questions:
What do I want, or what do I need to focus on now?
How can I achieve it? List them out in steps.
Why do I want it?

What skills and capabilities do I need to achieve it?

At this point in my life, what do I want?

What steps do I need to take to achieve them?

Prioritize the steps at the level of your passion

(Focus on the first 3)

You feel you're living and not existing.............. **Journal!**

You feel empty .... **journal!**

Your mind is disturbed................................ **journal!**

If you're confused, write down your thoughts.

DIARY

I love to write down what God says to me daily in my diary and my daily experience. Sometimes, we would like to share our daily experience with someone. Pick up your diary and write about your day, this is you giving yourself attention, and it results in loving yourself.

HOW TO ANSWER CLARITY QUESTIONS AND PLAN FOR YOUR DREAMS OR GOAL:
1. What do I want?

List as many things that come to your mind, don't leave back anything. Write exclusively.

Prioritize them as you feel they are essential and how you're passionate about them.

Pick the first three priorities

Pick the first 1

Make it clear and be specific now

For example, I want to become successful............. The subconscious mind can't work on this information, and it's too general, neither specific nor clear. You need to narrow it down for the brain to process. I want to become successful financially.

1. **HOW AM I GOING TO ACHIEVE IT?**
- Through investing in crypto, gold, and silver
- Through business [not specific or clear]

So, through business [oil and gas]

1. **BREAK EACH INTO STEPS TO ACHIEVE IT.**
- Crypto!

I will register for a course from the academy; I heard Betty talk about training on crypto. I will find out the price to start saving for the course.

- Silver!

I will search online [YouTube and Google] on how to start; I'll search for courses and webinars.

- Gold!

I will search online [YouTube, Facebook groups, and Google] on how to start, ask some friends, and search for courses and webinars.

- Oil and gas!

I will ask my friend's dad about it and do some findings online. I'll look out for seminars and conferences.

1. WHY DO YOU WANT IT?

I need a business to earn more money for investment. I need to invest to multiply my money, feed millions but thousands of students on scholarship, and achieve my luxury lifestyle. Your why must be compelling; if not, you won't be committed to it. Your 'why'' might be similar to those list above, but those are not compelling enough. What the reason you want to earn more money, get house......?

E. WHICH OF THE STEPS IN THE PLAN CAN YOU START TODAY?

I will call Betty today to ask about the academy again and the cost to get started.

I will search online to get a mentor or an academy to mentor me for silver and gold.

F. MAKE A MOVE TOWARDS YOUR PLAN DAILY.

Be intention to do something daily that moves you toward your goals.

JOURNAL DAILY:

It's essential to journal daily to update your plans; when you are conscious of the plans daily, you'll find out you do something that takes you closer to achieving your dreams.

· Set your alarm until your time is up, don't stand up.

· You can progress from 15 to 30mins daily and 1 hour.

G. TAKE MASSIVE ACTION:

Be uncomfortable with inaction. Take action daily.

H. STRUCK/UNSTUCK:

I don't know what to do again. Get a mentor or surround yourself with what can inspire you; you can also go for materials, watch videos on YouTube and register for a course online. Attend seminars, webinars, and more.

I. ARE YOU SCARED?

Does anything scare you? Are you bothered?

Courage is not the absence of fear but doing it anyway.

It's your turn to plan toward your dream or goals.

Get your pen. Remember,

"Don't let your learning lead to knowledge, let your learning lead to action." — Jim Rohn.

It's time to take action!!!

A. WHAT DO I WANT?

....

....

....

....

....

....

....

....

B. HOW AM I GOING TO ACHIEVE IT?

....

....

....

....

....

....

....

....

....

....

C. BREAK EACH INTO STEPS TO ACHIEVE IT?

....

....

....

....

....

....

....

....

....

....

D. WHY DO YOU WANT IT?

....
....
....
....
....
....
....
....
....
....

E. WHICH OF THE STEPS IN THE PLAN CAN YOU START TODAY?

....
....
....
....
....
....
....
....

F. WHAT MOVES ARE YOU MAKING TOWARDS YOUR PLAN TODAY?

....
....
....

MASTERY:

Principles govern life.

Regardless of who you are or where you are from, if you follow the right principles, you will get the right result. Mastery is the learning of a skill involving the spirit, soul & body. Everyone must go through the three levels of mastering to master any skill.

Three significant levels of mastery:

· Mental mastery

· Emotional mastery

· Physical mastery

MENTAL MASTERY:

Skills are internalized mentally; this is the level at which you'll understand the skills. No one will understand what you understand if you can't interpret it for them. It's the level of knowing the skills and becoming familiar with them. At this level, you know what you want and how to get it by watching videos, reading books, listening to podcasts, consumer training programs, seminars, and conferences.

Knowledge is potential power. Execution is power! -Tony Robbins.

Head knowledge is not enough.

EMOTIONAL MASTERY:

Skills are internalized emotionally at this level. Information without emotion is barely retained. *You have to repeat to create emotional mastery continually.*

At this level, you move from head knowledge to mind knowledge and start acting on the knowledge you have from level one.

Don't let your learning lead to knowledge. You'll become a fool. Let your learning lead to action, and then you'll become wealthy. -Tony Robbins.

PHYSICAL MASTERY:

Repetition is the mother of skill –Tony Robbins.

The skills are automatic at this level; you've repeated the mental and emotional skills enough that it has become a habit that expresses itself automatically. It's incredible who we can become and what we can do if we do something for a decade. Don't judge yourself too soon. Keep going.

"Mastery is not a function of genius or talent. It is a function of time and intense focus applied to a particular field of knowledge." — Robert Greene.

It's time to take action by being clear about what we want and setting goals.

Are you ready?

"A real decision is measured by the fact that you've taken a new action. If there's no action, you haven't truly decided." – *Tony Robbins*.

CHAPTER 4

COME OUT OF HIDING.

"Repetition is the mother of learning, the father of action, which makes it the architect of accomplishment." – Zig Ziglar

You have to be addicted to actions, not learning. You can take as many courses as you want, watch you tube videos, read books, attend conferences and seminars. If you don't take action, I mean massive action towards your goals, you won't see the desired result. You have to be addicted to taking action. Let inaction make you uncomfortable. Learning and not executing is like a man who has a product to sell. He goes to the market daily to learn how to sell and negotiate but never goes with his product. ***You can have the skills and capability and do nothing***. Remember, knowledge is not power, execution is power. You have to take action when it's convenient and inconvenient.

IDEAS

Dreams start with an idea in your mind, pictures in your head, and Imagination in your soul. Thus, these ideas inspire you and give your lives meaning. Having an idea and setting your goals towards it is life driven. When a man has nothing he's pursuing or working on, life becomes boring for such people. You indeed have a destiny and purpose but both change per season of your life. My purpose for this season might be to grow spiritually and also to mentor people spiritually while in the next season of my life, my purpose could be to teach people about financial freedom since destiny is an event that is inevitable. So, each time you obey your purpose per season, you fulfill your destiny. Destiny and purpose invariably change per season. But most times remains in the same specialty. Note; from the example above, the person keeps teaching about spirituality and finances, which indicates the person has teaching gift.

INTENTIONAL/UNINTENTIONAL:

Intentional idea:

These are ideas you brainstorm. If you want to start a business and need an idea about the business, you can brainstorm, pray, and consult people for ideas.

Unintentional idea:

These are ideas that keep showing up as pictures in your head, and you will keep imagining them. You see yourself doing it and you call them dreams or visions.

When an idea pops up in your head, you should be curious to know the purpose. Until you understand the purpose, you won't be motivated to execute the Idea. It's okay not to fully understand at first, but when you are conscious about knowing the purpose, it becomes more evident. Some ideas can stay in your head for months and years. If you don't question them to know the purpose. Sometimes, they reveal their purpose as time passes by.

To execute an idea, you have to know why.

Be clear and specific about your why.

Questions of Ideas

What is this Idea about?

How does this Idea impact my life?

How does this Idea impact others?

How does this impact you? Write in a sentence.

How does this impact others? Write in a sentence.

How to answer the ideas questions.

e.g., Idea; create a course on spirituality and finance for teenagers.

What's this Idea about? To educate the teenagers and expose them to spirituality and finance early during their secondary education.

How does this impact my life?

Being able to give the younger ones the skills and capability. I wish someone gave me to start my spiritual and financial journey early. This bring fulfillment and add to my source of income.

How does this impact others?

It will set a solid foundation for teenagers to start their spiritual and financial journey early in life. If they have the tools early, there is a high probability they will start early. I didn't have the tools early, so it held me back.

How does this impact you? Write in a sentence.

- Fulfillment from teaching the teenagers.
- Increase in finance

How does this impact others? Write in a sentence.

Basic knowledge to thrive spiritually and financially.

It's your turn to take action on the questions of ideas.

What's your Idea?

Note: just one Idea

....

....

....

....

....

What is this Idea about?

Write as much as you can; everything that pops in your head, whether it makes sense to you or not.

....
....
....
....
....
....
....

How does this Idea impact my life?

....
....
....
....
....
....

How does this Idea impact others?

....
....
....
....

How does this impact you? Write in a sentence.

....
....
....
....

How does this impact others? Write in a sentence.

....
....
....
....

Always remember your why should be compelling enough to keep pushing you. If it's just about you, your family, and making money, it's not compelling enough.

Congratulations, if you answer the previous questions, you are a step closer to birthing that idea.

RESEARCH:

When you're clear about the purpose of your Idea, then you can research. Note: your Idea gets clearer as you take the steps necessary to birth that idea.

FIRST QUESTION.......

WHAT DO I NEED TO ACHIEVE THIS?

List all the things you need to achieve the Idea.

To create a course;

- a camera,

- lightening [ring light]
- learn video editing/pay someone
- How to create a landing page
- List all that comes to your mind.

B. BREAK EACH OF THEM INTO STEPS TO ACHIEVE IT.

Camera
- I can't afford one now, but my phone can make a quality video.

OR
- I will talk to a friend or a colleague that has a camera if he can lend me for a while
- I'll speak to my parent to see if they can get me a camera
- I'll start saving to get a good phone and camera.
- How much will a good phone or camera cost?
-

To learn video editing:
- Learn from YouTube video
- How many megabytes will it cost me to watch more videos (location where the internet is limited)?
- Get a course to get results faster.
- How much will this course cost me?

List ways to achieve your goals and break them down into steps. If you get tired, close the book and come back later. But, don't stop or neglect for too long. Procrastinating to finish will

incur delay, and this will prevent you from achieving your goals.

EXECUTION:

You don't have to get all you need before you birth the Idea. When you can afford any of the things you need to execute the Idea, buy it. This send signal to the brain that you still want to execute the Idea. Both your soul and spirit will work together to make the Idea a reality. Be so conscious of all you need, and try to seize every opportunity that comes your way to achieve it. Plan on how to get the things you don't have. This can prompt an intentional idea to fund this Idea. Most people that birth their dreams will tell you they never had the enough money to fund their dreams. They had to get a job or start a business, and invest in funding their dreams. Stop waiting for a large sum of money to fund your dreams. You might wait forever. While waiting, you become less conscious of it. You know of the dream but are not conscious of it. Until you are consumed by your dreams and ideas in your head, you can't birth them.

MASSIVE ACTION.

Lisa Nichol said; **Action is the prescription for success.**

If you are tired of your life, start taking new and uncomfortable actions. Taking new and uncomfortable actions will lead you to an unrecognized positive life of your dreams. *Hoping and wishing makes you feel good, learning makes you feel closer and better, but action is what will get you the result. If you don't take action, you won't see the result you want.* Be addicted to taking action. This is the only way to change your life.

You can pray for many hours and speak in tongues daily, but God won't come down to take action for you. Your friend and family have a limit to which they can help you. It's your responsibility to take massive action to change your life. Anything that stops you from taking massive action stops you from achieving your dreams and goals. It is also stopping you from having the future you want.

Pain is inevitable, but suffering is a choice. Action is what puts suffering to perpetual sleep. Have you been the same person for so long? Start taking new actions. New actions will birth the change you want to see in your life, family, finances, and spiritual life. For things to change, you must change. For things to become better, you must be better. If you want to change your life, look for new answers. To get new answers, you have to ask new questions.

You can use fear as a motivation or a source of demotivation. If you're taking a new action, fear will show up because the brain is not used to the new activity you are about to execute. So, it will send the fear signal to explain that it's not used to the new command you are about to take. As you repeat the action, the brain gets used to it and won't send the fear signal with time.

Action is the antidote to fear

Consistency is an antidote to fear.

Result is an antidote to fear.

PERFECTION:

Perfection is an illusion, stop waiting for it. What you call perfection today won't be perfection in the next five years. It would be a mirage. Perfection is an excuse never to show up and take action. It's an excuse not to go all in. It's an excuse not to immerse yourself into the vision you're birthing. Focus on progress, not perfection. You have to keep working, make mistakes, correct yourself and keep going.

CERTAINTY/MOMENTUM

Momentum is the difference between success and failure. Emotions get us to start, momentum keeps us going, and certainty creates momentum. When you're certain about something, you'll put your all in and take action. You will see the result you want. But, when you're not certain, you don't go all in. you'll take a little action which will lead to a result you don't like.

Uncertainty = low self-confident = act small

You are born ready but not certain. You don't see a straight line in nature; you see up and down. Successful people have failed so much that they call it learning. When I'm not ready, that's when I'm ready. When I think I can't, then I must do it. Be willing to be uncertain, that's how you get the result you've never gotten before. You have to be immersed in getting the result you want, and hunger means you have decided not to settle for less.

When you go all in, you don't have a plan B. if you have a plan B, you dabble. Nothing works when you dabble. You must be willing to try as many times as possible till you get your desired result.

ENERGY:

When you sit to read for long, you most likely find yourself feeling a bit down. You might even tell yourself you're sad. When you say that, the body conforms to your confession. That moment, imagine you jump up unexpectedly, you will smile, and this will change your mood. What you do outwardly play a vital role in your energy.

Low energy; low-level emotion, negative taught, and low level taught.
High energy; high level of emotions, positive taught and high level taught.
Energy comes from habit. You're creators of your habits.

When you have nothing to hide, proof, defend, and protect, you're authentic or supreme self will show up, and you'll permit yourself to be in creation.

GIVE YOURSELF PERMISSION

You have to give yourself permission to take massive action and immerse yourself in your goals. To give yourself permission is the awareness of your inner being. Your soul and spirit understand what you are about to do. If your soul and spirit don't understand, you'll keep going back to the old pattern even though your brain is aware this is beyond your brain. It's about you tapping into your soul to draw out something new. When your inner being gets the message, execution becomes easy. There is a saying, "If you want to build an island, burn the boat." When your brain realizes there is no way out, it will find how to survive.

IMPOSTER SYNDROME

Imposter syndrome is a psychological occurrence in which an individual doubts their skills, talents, or accomplishments and has persistent internalized fear that they won't live up to expectations. It's when you believe negative stories in your head.

"No one cares about me."

"I can't do this."
 "I'm stupid."
"I don't have enough money to start."
"Who will buy from me?"
"Who will I sell to?"
"Who wants to listen to me?"
"Who will watch my videos on YouTube?"
"I don't think my handwriting is good enough."
"Being successful is hard."
"Things like this are not for people like me."

The stories you're telling yourself matters, the conversation going on in your head will inadvertently affect your belief system and result. If you don't believe right, you can't act right. What stories are you telling yourself that stop you from seeing the result?

Relationship:

....

....

....

Finances:

....

....

....

Career:

....

....

....

Spiritual:

....

....

....

Health:

....

....

....

NEGATIVE SELF TALK

You can't avoid them, but you can manage them. An increase in information helps to manage negative self-talk appropriately. Negative talk stems from negative experiences. It takes the right information or exposure to change negative self-talk. When you notice yourself talking negatively, pause and say the right thing. Don't lie to yourself. Tell the truth.

For instance,

- Marriage won't allow me to be the best version of myself.

Instead, you'll say,

I believe God has a man/woman who can accommodate my visions and anointing.

- Making money is difficult.

Making money is easy for me

- I will never be successful; no one in my family is ever successful.

I believe God will lead my path and direct me to success.

Write the stories you should be telling yourself to get the result you want

Relationship:

....

....

....

Finances:

....

....

....

Career:

....

....

....

Spiritually:

....

....

....

Health:

....

....

....

Read the lies and the truth for two days for each area together. On the third day, read out loud only the truth till your brain gets accustomed to the truth. These questions are called "Expose the lies"- by Lisa Nichol.

CUT OUT EVERY DISTRACTION

As you birth your idea, there will be distractions. Family members will show up to let you know what's not working, friends will be wondering what's happening, and some will be coming to you for advice. At the same time, some still expect you to show up as you do before. You can't keep serving everyone and everything you used to serve. You need space. You need to focus and get your priority right. To those that are close to you, let them know you're working on something new, and it requires total dedication. You have to let go of everything that may serve as distractions. Don't hold unto things that will serve as distractions, stop using your loved ones as an excuse.

Anything that prevents you from giving full attention to your goals is a distraction. One way to recognize distractions is that they demand immediate attention. You have to learn to prioritize and recognize your need from your want. Remember, limiting belief sounds like excuse. Cut off as many or any form of distraction.

Distractions are like a heavy weight that holds you back. Imagine someone in a race and keep looking back or left and right. Every time he looks around, he loses focus and misses a step.

In the process of birthing your dream, you would become a new person. This new version of you can serve your family, friends, spouse, colleagues, and every other person better. To serve them better, you must become an improved version of yourself. To improve yourself, they have to excuse you; give you the time and space you need. You have to explain and help them understand your current season. If they don't understand now, they will understand later. But you have to save yourself first and come back to save them. If you don't rescue yourself first, you will all remain at that same level. Cut off every form of distraction to rescue your future self.

FAMILY:

I love you, but I have a dream to bring to life. I have a picture in my head to make a reality. I can't stay with you to make you comfortable, but I will be back. Say that to people that need to hear it. I love you, but I need my space and time. If I can't have that, I have to go. I will be back. My soul is screaming to soar. It's screaming, don't hold me back. Set me free. Let me soar! Tell yourself this season, I'm going to master myself.

When our races are all done on earth, we shall stand before God, and one thing is sure, we are going to give account for the assignment he committed into our hands while we are alive.

Nothing like, "My husband, my wife, my parent, my friends, finances, or ignorance didn't allow me to execute them, there will be no room for excuses, neither will there be room for failure.

ENVIRONMENT:

Don't allow your background put your back on the ground – Frank Edward.

It's not about your background but your future address. Where do you want to go? Avoid self-pity. If I didn't see my daddy smoke, I wouldn't smoke, you might see you dad do it, but it's your choice to accept and express it. It's all about your choice. You might grow up in a dysfunctional family, or you might grow up being traumatized, but it's not the event that happens that matters but your interpretation of the event. Nothing has meaning except the meaning you give to it. What meaning are you giving your background?

Let's expose some lies we tell ourselves:

My dad cheated on my mum.

My first boyfriend cheated on me.

I'm not interested in marriage, all men are cheaters.

You can conclude all men are cheaters because these two men cheated.

Question are all men cheaters? No.

Truth; Not all men cheat.

What are the lies from your background that affects you in finance?

No one in my family ever has up to 5000 dollars in their account. I don't think I can too.

What's the truth? I can have 5000 dollars in my account, but it will require me not to handle money the way my family does.

CAREER:

If you don't study medicine, law, or engineering, it will be difficult for you to become successful.

Truth: I can be financially free when I'm mentored by those who are financially free.

SPIRITUAL:

If you have a challenge, it's because you're not praying enough

Truth: Because I have a relationship with God doesn't mean I can't have challenges.

HEALTH: I just can't stop eating late at night. I think I inherit it from my home.

Truth: I can stop eating late at night. I deserve good health.

Relationship:

....

....

....

Finances:

....

....

....

Career:

....
....
....

Spiritual:

....
....
....

Health:

....
....
....

What's the truth?

Relationship:

....
....
....

Finances:

....
....
....

Career:

....
....
....

Spiritual:

....

....

....

Health:

....

....

....

COMPANY.

The company you keep and the people you share your dreams with matters. They can help strengthen your dreams or act otherwise. In transition season, there is an isolation phase where you experience inner conversation than outer conversation. The isolation phase can be lonely, but you have to stay in your head and focus on your dreams and goals. Don't let loneliness prevent you from rescuing your future.

You can have all the knowledge you need to birth your dreams, but your environment and company influence might not permit you to practice. When you don't practice, your morale to take action goes down. When you don't take action, you can't see your desired result.

The people you're surrounded with can generate a strong influence on you and probably hold you hostage so that you don't get to practice what you've learned. You have to be around those that tell you the truth about yourself, believe in you, motivate you for success, and support you in achieving your goals.

Sometimes, the people that surround you drain you. They are close to you, but you have to be selfish for you to be able to birth your dreams. Selfishness is good as far as this concept is concerned. If perhaps it will allow you to have the time and space to become a better you. You should prioritize your time and give time to things that are important to you, such as family, work, and self. When it's your personal time, it's okay to be selfish with it.

Let's expose our company:
1. Are your companies draining you? **Yes or No**
2. Is this person/relationship moving me forward or backward? **YES/ NO**
3. Do I have enough time for myself? **YES/NO**

COURAGE:

Being courageous is not the lack of fear, but you do it anyway. Fear will show up every time you are about to take a new step. Our brain is programmed to help us survive. So, every time you are about to do what the brain doesn't have a record of, it sends the fear signal that expresses itself through your emotions. You feel uncomfortable. You start procrastinating. You say to yourself
"I will do it later."
"I don't feel like doing it now."
You give all sorts of excuses. Remember, limiting belief sound like excuse. You make excuse and not take action. Learn to question all the stories you tell yourself every time you want to take action.

Why can't I do it now? Is it true I don't feel like doing it, or am I just scared? When you know the root of the excuse, you can overcome the power of the effect. Then tell yourself a new story to empower and support you to take action. If you don't feel like doing it now, then you must. You must learn to manage and control yourself through the conversations you have with yourself.

PROCRASTINATION:

Greg Erhabor said, "Procrastination is the grave in which opportunities are buried. It is not just the thief of time; it is the thief of destiny. Procrastination is deferring what you should do today till tomorrow. Procrastination is postponing your success till another day. When you delay in your responsibilities, you are setting yourself up for failure. What you have to do, do it quickly."

If you don't want your future to look like your yesterday, you have to do away with Procrastination. If you don't feel like doing it, then you must do it! I will do it tomorrow, then you have to do it today. Don't let Procrastination steal your dream life. Each time you procrastinate, you will always come back to meet it undone. Hence, continuous Procrastination can lead to frustration that makes us neglect our dreams. To achieve our dream,you have to learn to manage negative self-talk and learn to disempower our limiting beliefs. If not, you'll find yourself procrastinating and delaying the birthing of your dreams.

CONFIDENCE:

Confidence is not something you are born with, you do things that create self-confidence. Repetition of habit can increase or decrease your self-confidence. To increase your self-confidence, you have to recognize what decreases your self-confidence. Some people would say, "Work hard on your weaknesses" why waste time working hard on your weaknesses when you can empower your strength; your strength will overcome your weaknesses.

What are the things that diminish your self-confidence on the inside?

Do you feel Unworthy?

Do you doubt yourself?

Question your feelings to disempower them.

FAILURE/FEAR:

Every setback is a stronger comeback – Joel Osteen.

You have to be okay to fail a lot of time to be successful; if you want to become successful, you have to be neutral to failure and realize failure is part of the process to success. Thomas Edison failed one thousand times before he arrived at the solution that forever changed the world. On the journey of birthing your dreams, failure is inevitable. You have to be okay with it and see it as a springboard for success. Every time you want to take a new step, fear is inevitable. It's a sign the brain will send to you, which means; I'm not familiar with this. Be courageous and comfortable with being afraid. Take massive action regardless.

DREAM REQUIRES SACRIFICE

"Understand there is a price to be paid for achieving anything of significance. You must be willing to pay the price." John Wooten.

If a phone costs $1500 and you're willing to pay $1500, you are indirectly saying you value the phone more than your $1500. So, it's okay to let go of it to have the phone you desire. It's the same with your dreams. How much are you willing to pay for your dreams?

Dreams are free, but the journey is not. Your dream will cost you more money and time than you imagine. It will cost you your friends, family, and sometimes your spouse. The closest people to you will criticize your dream.
Are you willing to pay the price for your dream?
Are you willing to let go of weekend parties and social gatherings with friends?
Are you willing to do the things you've never done before?
Are you willing to be uncomfortable for a while?

Chasing your dreams requires discipline, courage, and commitment.
It requires you to face your fears. Say what you've never said before.
Are you willing to pay the price for your dream?

"If the first thing that we've chosen to do is to calculate the cost, we've already betrayed the dream." - **Craig D. Lounsbrough**.

When you sign up for your dream, sign up for the inconvenience too. It's not going to be easy, but it will worth it. Your dreams won't happen easily or as quickly as you might want them to. Are you willing to be inconvenient for a while to achieve your dream? Pursuing your dreams will not be a stroll in the park for you—the reason many never achieve their dreams. The journey is difficult and would force you to learn along the way. You will be uncertain many times. Your life can't continue to live your old life, if you are going to chase your dreams. You have to change for your dream to become a reality.

You underestimate the cost of your dreams. Some dreams take years to achieve. Are you willing to be married and committed to your dream? Dream takes time, money, energy, and much more. That's the reason you have to plan now and start working on it today.

DISPLAY YOUR GIFT:

Many times, you wait on people to help and give you platforms to display your gifts. Social media and YouTube allow you display your gifts. Don't wait on people! You have to be okay with what you have. It doesn't have to be perfect. It just has to impact lives. You have to stop thinking about yourself but those that your gift will impact. It's not about you but about the people the gift will impact. Always remember, every master was once a student.

REPETITION

I listened to Tyler Perry tell a story of how he got people to drill a well in his company premises. They tried the first time, no water. He had to pay the money even though they didn't get water. He called them the second time, and in the same situation the third time, he called them and said, until you reach water, don't stop digging. Guess what? They found water just 2 meters away.

If you're not convinced about what you want, you'll back out too soon. You don't get the desired result when you dabble. You have to be all in. if you have plan B, you're not all in. The mindset that births the desired result is a mind that sticks to one plan and is flexible in its approach to the plan. Change plan to achieve the dream as many times as possible.

Most ideas don't work out the first time. Make mistakes, correct them fast and keep moving. That is what is called fail forward. Work hard and smartly. Follow your mentor's procedure. You can't neglect any step on the journey to success. If not, you won't be able to replicate the success.

If you think you've tried your best and yet, the result is a deadlock. You can genuinely ask yourself, have I tried all I know?

Get mentors to coach you for the desired result, don't give up too quickly. Be determined not to back out till you've gotten your desired result. Stay in the game till you get the desired result. If you don't get tough mentally, you won't be able to withstand the demand of success.

I'M TIRED/ I'M STUCK

On the journey to achieve your goals, you can fag out, get tired, and stuck. Relax and quickly remember why you started in the first place. At this point, you have to 'RE' do all you've done.

RE-commit

RE-dedicate

RE-align

RE- design

RE-organize

RE-set

RE-motivate/

RE- inspire

Remember, the journey is not an easy one, but it is worth it. No doubt, you will get stuck at one point or the other. It shows you're on the right path, but get unstuck, get yourself to "RE" the question you want to ask yourself is, what do I need to focus on now?

What do I need to focus on now?

Maximum of 3lists

....

....

....

Prioritize them and arrange in order of urgency.

....

....

....

Pick the first one and focus on that only for now.

....

What's distracting you?

....

....

....

If what's distracting you is what you have to do, how can you manage the distractions? Pick each distraction and write under it how to manage it.

....

....

....

What do you need to help you focus more?
e.g., inspiring videos on the current goals.

....

....

....

List 7 things you are proud of since you started working on this goal.

....

....

....

....

....

....

....

EXERCISE

The journey to achieve your goal will demand strength from your spirit, soul, and body.

You have to feed your spirit, soul, and body.

Feed and strengthen your mind every day

Take time off daily, maybe 30min [less or more], to be your time of learning something new. Let it be your "ME" time. Let it be the time you recharge and improve yourself to become a better person. Read something new daily. New information can help you RE-strategize better and move faster. You can't neglect to learn on the journey of birthing your goals.

Tony Robbins said, "We are all equal in spirit and soul but not in the marketplace. Value distinguishes us in the marketplace."

Feed and strengthen your body

When you exercise, the brain secretes some hormones;

Dopamine

Serotonin

GABA [Gamma Amino Butyric Acid]

After the day's activity or sitting for a long time, you might be tired and stressed. Try to sleep but can't due to body pain. Exercise might help you.

DOPAMINE HORMONE:

The **dopamine hormone** is also called the **feeling good hormone.** When you exercise, dopamine is secreted, and it gives a feeling of euphoria [Intense excitement and happiness], bliss [Great joy], motivation, and concentration. Dopamine plays a vital role in the movement, sleep, learning, mood, memory, and attention.

SEROTONIN:

This hormone helps in mood stabilization and in helping one feel a sense of well-being and happiness. It plays a vital role in sleeping, digestion, reward, eating, memory and learning. Little of this hormone is in the brain and is associated with depression and anxiety.

GABA [GAMMA AMINO BUTYRIC ACID]

When GABA is secreted, it blocks specific signals in the brain that reduces fear, anxiety, and stress.

When you feel down and weak………. Exercise

Depressed? ………………Exercise

Anxiety? ……………………..Exercise

Not getting good sleep ?…………… Exercise

You can exercise in the morning and make the evening for long walk. Walks are as good as exercise. Exercise is essential. It keeps you focus, makes you feel good, stabilizes your mood, and reduces your stress, fear, and anxiety.

FEED YOUR SPIRIT:

Sharing time with your manufacturer will grant you peace that surpasses all human understanding. You experience rest. You receive revelations that constantly keep you inspired. Your faith grow to believe your goals are achievable.

MARCO AND MICRO WIN.

"Learn to celebrate your success; else failure will celebrate you as an unsung hero" — Dr.P.S. Jagadeesh Kumar.

The journey of achieving your big goals might take days, months, or years. To prevent you from getting demotivated, celebrating your wins is essential. Imagine someone hitting the gym daily for 2weeks, the desired result might not be visible, but the person is not the same anymore.

When you track your small wins every day and weekly, it will boost your motivation which will in turn, build your self-confidence. When next you set a goal, you can leverage on the past result. If you could achieve your last goal, then you can do this. As you reward yourself, the feel-good hormone is created to motivate you to do more. When you're motivated, you'll want to take more action.

CELEBRATE YOUR WINS

You must acknowledge your progress and not perfection. If you don't feel good about your work, even if you've not arrived at the desired result. You won't be happy. When you are not happy, nothing works.

You must write down your wins; when you write down your wins, you can always go back to them when you're down and demotivated. Write down your wins, and staring at them makes you feel good and boost your self-confidence. Just as you have a vision board, have a win board where you can always see the things you've accomplished. So, on days you're down, you can quickly go and stare at them.

Take a day off; Take time to relax. It keeps you refreshed. You get to focus on other things like spending time with your loved ones. Doing things you enjoy, and has a way it increases your creative level and makes you feel relaxed so you can focus better when you're back at work.

Gift yourself: learn to reward yourself with things that excite you to do better. It doesn't have to be expensive.

Share your wins with others; sharing your wins has a way it boost your self-confidence, resulting in you working more to get the bigger wins. You may likely be selective with whom you share your small wins. You might share with people you know and trust personally and that support you and care about your dream. When you, therefore, have your big wins, you can invite everyone and make it an event.

Acknowledge God; go to God with sincere gratitude in your heart. You can't guarantee you will wake up tomorrow morning. This is to remind us that we don't own our lives. Be grateful for the privilege to be alive, the strength to work on your projects, and the inspiration and ideas. Many have goals but got stuck on how to make them a reality. you are already on the journey to make it happen, so you should be grateful to God. You can start by saying, "God, thank you for all you have done. Thank you for your inspiration and strength to work on this goal. With your help, I know this goal will be a reality. Thank you for watching out for me when I'm not even aware. Thank you for your invisible hand that command impressive results on this project".

DON'T USE GOD AS AN EXCUSE

I serve people who have a prayer list full of things God doesn't do. Half of the things they're asking God to do are tables and chairs, and He does trees. If they could catch what I'm talking about, we could go to pray about stuff that matters.

        –T.D Jakes.

Many waits for God to do what they are meant to do like to pay their bills, make their marriage work, give them the lifestyle they want, and make their business grow. But all these are your responsibilities. God will never fail in His responsibility, but many times, we fail in our responsibilities and charge the blame on God. If you pray for an increase in your finance, God will inspire you and grant your ideas and strategies that can help you grow in your finance. That is His part; , therefore, your responsibility to get a related course, books, videos, and mentors that can help you. God won't learn the skills and capability for you, God won't plan your goals for you, but He will direct your steps.

Your business is not growing the way you want. It's great to pray and put your trust in God. Also, get a coach to help you out. Financial coaching for instance is essential in other for you to be able to grow or skyrocket your income. Get them to help you.

I have realized you can pray for a solution in any area of life, and God tell you the solution, but if your mind doesn't

understand what God is saying to you, you will still be in the same condition.

It will still come down to the level of your mind. God walk with you at the level of your minds. God will send people to help you come across information that can help. Most times, many needs a prophecy or the necessity to hear from their pastors before they can believe.

God has given you a vision, and you are expecting Him to implement it. How you know you're waiting on God is that you do nothing about the vision he has shared with you, No plan. Not learning the skills and capability to make that vision a reality. If this happens, do you expect Him to trust you with more visions? It's against the law of management.

Worthy of note is the fact that God doesn't control you, nor does He force you to do anything out of your will. When God gives, He doesn't take back. He gave you free will, and with our free will, we get to decide if we'll obey Him or not. He doesn't choose for you; He only advised you on what to do—the same with marriage. God will present your partner to you but won't force you to choose them.

Not everything that happens is **God's will.** The only place where everything that happens is **God's will is** in heaven. The earth has been given to man to subdue. God controls heaven. Men control the earth. That's big for a religious mind to accept. But, it's the truth. Reasons we pray is to enforce **God's will** here on earth. The danger of words like "God is in control" and "Whatever happens is God's will" is what makes you blame God and not take ownership; this results in you not taking full responsibility. Until you start taking full responsibility for your lives, you can't implement destiny or live your best life.

QUESTIONS

If you don't manage your anger and your marriage fails, is that God in control?

If you don't learn time management and do not meet up with your duties at work, is that God in control?

If you have a terrible relationship with money, money doesn't stay in your hand for too long that you fall short of paying your bills. Is that God in control? You have outgrown your mindset and can't make more money. Is that God in control?

Yes, He's awe-inspiring, miraculous and mysterious, all-knowing, sovereignty, which means. At the same time, you make your choices, and they have consequences.

GOD IS MIRAULOUS, NOT A MAGICIAN

You see miracles happen, but you simply don't understand the requirement. You behave as God will act without your consent, in most cases you neglect your responsibilities. You are partners with God for the things He wants to do here on earth. God is a moral God. He wants you to take action and be aggressive about issues. When God says to move, and you don't move, you'll miss the miracle and don't make it look like God had failed you when He asked you to move,

Faith is great! But many forget faith requires action. We've been told to praise and pray our ways out of situations, but doing the work is not emphasized. God will send you a challenge so you can change your perspective and come out of your comfort zone. You have to be tired of being in the same problem for too long. Be tired of going through the same old problem, and be tired of complaining. If you're calling on God and the situation is not changing, it's a sign God is using it to move you. Don't give up too quickly.

While you're waiting on God, God is waiting on you to do something about the situation. We don't need to appease God before He gives us what we need. God loves you beyond watching you appease Him before He blesses you. Many have cried for so long. Your tears don't move God and won't change anything until you make a move. Then, God will move with you. If a child doesn't open their arms to be lifted, it will be challenging to carry the child, even though the child needs help. It's the same with God and us. God needs your permission to take action.

CHAPTER 5

FUND YOUR DREAM

Pivot because the world into which you were born no longer exists
–Cindy Trimm

To make your dream a reality, you need to get the right and appropriate information. You need to shift your mindset; this will enlighten you on what to do and get you to take massive action. Trial and error is not the best way to achieve your goals. Paying mentors for speed is how you get ahead and achieve your goals faster. As you work on your goals, you need a house over your head, keep the light on, access to the internet, food to keep you alive, and water to sustain you. You need to attend seminars and conferences and buy course materials and other materials essential to make your goal a reality. For all these to happen, you need money.

Living your dream life and achieving your goals will cost you more money than you think. Many destinies are stagnant because the mind can't see money. To bring to reality the pictures in your head, it is a necessity you learn how to finance your ideas and monetize their idea.

The world is structured in a way that money is central to all things in life, and so there is nothing so significant, great, and successful that does not require money. Many people shy away from talking about money. If you shy from talking about money, you won't have it. It's what you talk about, learn about and take action towards that you'll achieve. If you have to get your desired result towards money, you have to learn about it, talk about it and surround yourself with those who talk about it and possess it. Always remember, your finance is your responsibility.

NEW AGE

The only thing constant is change. Change is inevitable. Change happens to everyone and everything, including wealth creation. Over the years, we have seen a revolution in how people's work has changed significantly. Only those who are conscious of it learn to adapt fast, benefit from the revolution and get ahead financially in their generation.

AGRARIAN AGE

This is also known as the Neolithic age or agricultural age. In this age, the primary source of wealth was the cultivation of land (farming). Many societies focus on food production and land. Most people work on the land preceding the agrarian age were hunter-gatherers. At this age, most people worked for themselves and acknowledged creativity. People reach out to you more if you have a different design than they have. Many people were into farming, crafts, and merchants. According to Wikipedia, this age started around 6800 BCE in East Asia. This age transitioned into the industrial age.

INDUSTRIAL AGE:

This revolution began in Great Britain around 1760 and encompassed the changes in economic and social organization. It was the replacement of hand tools with machines. As people created machines to help them work faster and better, machines became an essential part of life. It was the age when most people were factory workers; creative thought was not encouraged as this could lead to dismissal from work. Factory owners were considered wealthy, and few people who couldn't afford machines worked for themselves.

INFORMATION AGE:
This is known as the computer age, digital age, or new media age. It's known as "The modern age where information has become a commodity that is quickly and widely disseminated and easily available, especially through the use of computer technology." [Merriam Webster].

People from the industrial age grew frustrated from their idea not being expressed. Because of the way they were treated, union trade was formed to ensure better working conditions. Information technology makes it easier and cheaper to work for oneself. Those who seek out new information are the ones who constantly succeed in the informative age, and this age encourages creativity and constant learning. Ideas are encouraged in the workplace in this era; one must be thinking of new ideas to be the best at their workplace.

Every time revolution happens, there is a lot of money to be made. Critics don't see the opportunity, but the analyzers do. If an analyzer takes massive action, he will get ahead in the next wave of wealth. When you study history, you'll realize it's the same pattern playing out in different scenarios. Still, the same principle can be used, which is to get educated about what's going on, seize the opportunity and take massive actions.

REVOLUTION:

As Eric Hoffer once said, "In times of change, learners inherit the earth, while the learned find themselves beautifully equipped to deal with a world that no longer exists."

Those that fail to revolutionize become left out of the new opportunities because they continue to think the old way. They know the old way they do things is not yielding results as it should, but they continue to do it; because they are not aware it's a new era. Many become frustrated, weak in their mind, and left with no choice but to get out of business. Some even think it's a spiritual problem and would pray as much as they can.

It's a new era. Those that have recognized the new age and made use of the opportunity have created wealth over time.

In the Agrarian Age, the rich were the monarchs and the nobles. If you were not born into this group, you were an outsider with little chance of becoming one of them.

During the industrial age, Wealth shifted from agricultural land to real estate; Wealth shifted from farm owners to buildings on the farmland. Farmers that didn't pivot had to work harder to survive.

The industrial age was when those not born noble had the opportunity to become rich and powerful. It was the first wave of wealth creation. It's when wealth giants like Andrew Carnegie, John D. Rockefeller, and Henry Ford became billionaires. Andrew Carnegie became a billionaire dominating the steel industry in the

US. John D. Rockefeller became a billionaire through his dominance in the oil and railroad industry. Henry Ford became a billionaire by creating the first automobile that middle-class Americans could afford; he converted the automobile from an expensive curiosity into accessibility.

INFORMATION AGE:

In this age, Quality and timely information help to build wealth. We find the wealth giants like Bill Gates, Michael Dell, Mark Zuckerberg, Jeff Bezos, and Elon Musk. In this era, the idea of hard work is not the same as it was in the agrarian and industrial age. It's not about working hard but working right and smart through business and investment.

STRUCK IN PAST AGE:

Go to school, get good grades and get a good job. If this statement is made in the industrial age, it's excellent, but if this is said to you today, it is not wise advice to take. Revolution has taken place. Yet! Parents born in the industrial era try to talk their children into obeying the industrial age rules. It's the age to encourage them to learn skills. That is what gets people money today, not grades, and this is why teenagers can be a millionaire by pressing their phones from home.

An economic expert who accurately predicted some of the things that might likely happen post- Covid – 19, he went further to provide insight on the aftermath of the Russia – Ukraine war. In all he said, he projected into the future to say. In Nigeria, for instance, in the next decade years, a university certificate will amount to nothing. He opined that the young ones should concentrate on skill acquisitions and entrepreneurship even though education is the bedrock of all.

Yet, projecting into the future and with the trajectory of events in this part of the world, entrepreneurship and skill acquisition will be the major trend for financial stability in the nearest future. In sincerity, it is evident that based on the technological advancement of the world generally, in most cases, machines have taken over some of the position's men should occupy, and so what is simply needed is the employment of few that can operate the machine. For instance, the banking system does not need as many employees as it used to have in the past years. The reason for this is technological advancement. No doubt, situations will yet continue like this. So it is far crucial for you to be able to discover yourself incisively and to plan on the aspect of skill acquisition and entrepreneurship. At the same time, education must remain an underlying factor.

Revolutionize to the present age by educating yourself about what's going on around you. If not, you will become rejected and unqualified. If you are in your teenage years or you're in your twenties or thirties, learning a skill is a necessity. It's a proper way of attaining financial stamina in the future.

HISTORY REPEATS ITSELF.

If you study the history of money from the first wave of wealth to the second, you would realize history repeated itself. But only those who study history and understand it can seize the opportunity when it shows up.

There have always been recessions and depressions. With the few years, I have spent on earth, I have never heard a price of a thing dropdown. It's always going up. Those who have studied history always prepare themselves to prosper whichever way the economy goes.

If history is any indicator, a person who lives to the age of 75 should anticipate going through one depression and two major recessions during their lifetime. - Roberts Kiyosaki.

RECESSION VERSUS DEPRESSION:

A recession is a normal part of the business cycle, it comes when there is an economic decline that lasts for two quarters, and the economic growth will slow down for several quarters before it turns negative.

INDICATORS

The unemployment rate will drop too low

People can't pay their loans

Oil price spikes

Stock market crashes

Decrease home prices and sales

Rising interest rate

Deflation

Depression is the drastic fall in economic activity that last for years rather than several quarters. It can be longer than a year, and it's more destructive. You'll know the economy is in depression if the indicator of recession last more than a year.

THE GREAT RECESSION:

The great recession is the economic collapse that happened from December 2007 to June 2009; this collapse occurred for nineteen months. It was triggered by the bursting of the real estate bubble; house bubbles start with an increase in house price due to high demand, and at some points, demand decreases or stagnates at the same time supply increases, resulting in a sharp drop in prices called bursting. Real estate bursting took place 2005-2006, then the global financial rises followed and lasted till 2009.

THE GREAT DEPRESSION:

The great depression was experienced in the US in 1929 and continued till the year 1930. It was a severe global economic breakdown which was considered the most prolonged and deepest economic downturn of the 20th century that swept the entire globe, triggered by a significant fall in stock prices in the US.

HISTORY IS A GUIDE:

Suppose you learn from history and take it as a guide. In that case, you will prepare for the recession and depression ahead, and this will give you an edge economically regardless of which direction the economy goes.

FUND YOUR DREAM:

"Most people think about having a better life, they think about being financially independent, they think about living their dreams, but the level of action is not in alignment with their thoughts. When you align your actions with your thoughts, the results are inevitable." – Lisa Nichols.

Lisa Nichols is one of the world's most requested motivational speakers and transformational coaches. Lisa grew up in a family that could afford her basic need but was always out of money before the month's end. At 28, Lisa was a single mother with a son of about eight months with barely any income, qualifying her for public assistance. One day she needed nappies for her son; she went to the ATM and had only $11.42 left in her bank account. She placed her hand on her son's tummy, and she said, "Jelani. Today will be the last time something like this happens. It was the turnaround moment for her.

"Everyone said invest in yourself first, write yourself a cheque, invest in your future, invest in your education," "Everyone kept saying invest, invest, invest, and I just started doing it." – Lisa Nichols.

Over the next few years, Lisa started reading books, attending entrepreneur conferences, getting a job and started saving. When her son was 3, she wrote her first cheque for $110 and deposited it into a savings account. Every two weeks, she wrote herself a cheque and ensured it was 5% more than the last cheque. She wrote on it, "Funding my dream," even though she didn't know what the dream was. She wanted to speak and inspire people. She knew it would cost her money to pay for mentorship to attend seminars and workshops.

Lisa Nichols got a second job to help her save more money and cut down on extra expenses. She said, "I wrote myself a cheque for three and a half years. I stopped getting my nails done, and I stopped getting my hair done, I stopped going out for dinners, I stopped taking my son to McDonald's, and I stopped going out dancing with my cousins. I sold my newer cars; I bought an older car. I moved out of my three-bedroom house. I moved in and became roommates with my friend. I was willing to inconvenient myself to keep writing bigger and bigger cheque.

Ms. Nichols wrote herself a cheque every 2weeks for three and half years. To prevent her from the trap of spending the money, she didn't open her bank statement. The day she went to the bank and was told she had $62500 to fund her dream. She said no! That can't be my money; she called her account number for them again. The cashier replied, "Ms. Nichols, that's your balance; she was surprised. She said ''no one in my family has ever had $5000 in their account.''

At some point, her family taught she was crazy or on drugs because she wasn't going out and socializing, but noticed she wasn't skinny. She wanted to be excellent and end every sentence from each speaker. This resulted in her attending the same conference 42 times.

Trainings cost money. She could afford it because she had prepared for it. She also pay someone to take care of her son during her trainings. Sometimes might pay for hotel; she was willing to be inconvenient till she achieved her goal.

Today, Lisa is CEO of "Motivate the Masses," which provides personal and business development training programs through coaching, courses, and speaking engagement. It was founded in 1998, went public in 2013, and is now on the NASDAQ stock exchange. Her global platform has reached nearly an 80million people. Through her nonprofit foundation motivating the teen spirit, she has touched the lives of over 270,000 teens, prevented over 3800 teen suicides, supported 2,500 dropouts in returning to school, and has helped thousands reunite with families.

Lisa is a noted media personality who has appeared on Oprah Winfrey's show, the today show, Dr. Phil show, the Steve Harvey Show, and many more. She is a featured teacher in the movie "The Secret" and the book with the same name, which has sold over 30 million copies worldwide. Once again, I ask you, "Are you willing to pay the price for your dream life?" Your dreams are valid. God didn't give you an inferior destiny, but you have an inferior destiny if you don't prepare well.

SAVING:

Before you start saving, you have to be clear on WHY you're saving.

Many have heard about saving, so they start saving. Along the line, get tired and stop saving, withdraw all the money and spend on daily needs or look sophisticated at a friend's party – "Pepper them gangs" (slang in Nigeria). They want the latest designer bag, perfume, watch, and so on.

When you are clear about why you're saving, you'll be motivated to keep saving and save more money. If you have a dream and you're not sure exactly what the dream is, it's going to cost you: I tell you, it will cost you more money than you imagine. The earlier you start saving to fund your dreams, the better. You will need to pay mentors for speed, buy books to read, listen to videos on YouTube, pay house rent and utility bills, and get courses, workshops, masterminds, and conferences.

PAY YOURSELF FIRST

The statement "Pay yourself first" comes from George Clason's book, "Richest Man in Babylon." If you are starting your financial journey or you are on the journey, one of the insightful books to read is the "Richest Man in Babylon." you pay many people but not yourself. You pay your landlords, utility bills, and groceries. But not yourself. Hence, your expenses are someone's income.

If you are a salary earner, self-employed, or you get allowances from the parent or husband. Pay yourself before paying others. Most people will respond; I won't have enough. Yes! There is never enough money until you work on your mind to see enough money.

Money is an idea, a means of exchange. Every time you give money away, what you're saying is, **you value what you want to buy than your money.** When you hear them tell you to pay them their money, pay yourself first. Your emotion is the first thing that responds, and the brain asks you how you will survive. If more money will solve that problem, getting a second job should. Most time, people get a second job and still find themselves sinking into debt more than ever. Why? Because they have not trained their minds to see money, until you train yourself to focus on your need and not want, you will keep buying what you want rather than your need.

On the journey to find your dream, buying your want will keep you on the journey more than you can imagine. Are you saying I should not enjoy my life? What I'm saying is, if you don't want to be on the journey of achieving your dream forever, you have to cut expenses. You have to be willing to be inconvenient for a while.

Remember what Lisa said, "I stopped getting my nails done, I stopped getting my hair done, I stopped going out for dinners, I stopped taking my son to McDonald's, I stopped going out dancing with my cousins. I sold my newer car; I bought an older car. I moved out of my three-bedroom house, I moved in,

and I became roommates with my friend. I was willing to inconvenient myself to keep writing bigger and bigger cheques."

Every penny counts on the journey to fund your dreams. Pennies make a dollar. One dollar spent on want will compound one day to 1000 dollars spent on wants. Until 1 dollar becomes important to you; you haven't recognized your need from want. If you're still wondering what the difference between need and want is, here they are:

NEED/WANT:
Need is anything essential for your survival, like food, cloth, or house, while a want is anything non-essential for the basic need for survival but a person desires to have. E.g., expensive cloth, living in a three-bedroom apartment all by yourself, to eat at fancy restaurants are all sequel to needs, not necessarily wants. Hence, needs and want differs from one person to another, as everyone is not on the same financial level. A person might want the car and another need a car.

Wants are significant but are you willing to delay the gratification of your wants for a while to achieve your dream life? Are you willing to be inconvenient for a while to achieve your dream life? Are you willing to overcome peer group influence and mind your business? Your dream life requires you to be inconvenient for a while.

Don't just sign up for your dream; sign up for the inconvenience too. Your dream life will cost you more than you could ever imagine. Are you willing to pay the price to make your dream a reality? It's like a pregnant woman that carries a baby for nine months; while on this journey, she feels pain and discomfort on many occasions, but when she remembers the result, she is encouraged to continue the journey. The reason you have to be clear about the result you want before you start saving, you might get tired at some point, but when you remember the result, you can quickly gain momentum back to keep going.

Ask yourself before saving

Why am I saving?

How long am I saving?

What's the goal amount before withdrawing?

What am I using the money for when I withdraw?

If you're still not clear on what to use your savings for, don't withdraw. If you are saving to fund your dreams, then the end goal should be one of the two options or both.

Invest in yourself; get the knowledge you need from mentors, courses, workshops, and conferences

Or

Multiply the money through business or investment

INVESTMENT VEHICLES

There are many vehicles; we have bicycles, cars, trucks, buses, airplanes, ships, boats, and so on. Where you are going will determine what type of vehicle you use. If you plan to arrive Nigeria from America in the next 24 hours, the best vehicle to gets you the result is an airplane. You won't want to get into a ship if you have to be in Nigeria within 24 hours. You can make the right decision because you are clear about where you are and where you want to be.

When you arrive to Lagos, Nigeria, and depart to Abuja, you can decide to go by air or road. If you want to appreciate the country, you can go by road using a private car or public bus. If you have to be in Abuja in the next 4 hours, the airplane is the most appropriate means of transportation.

A single person may not need a 9seater wagon, but a family of 5 would need one. A farmer would instead pick a truck than a two-seater sports car. So, you pick the vehicles you want, considering where you are and your needs. Vehicles vary from one person to another based on needs.

It's the same with investment. There are many vehicles to get you from where you are financial to where you want to be. No vehicle is better than the other; the lower the risk, the lower the return, the higher the risk, and the higher the return. So, you have to pick the one suitable for your plan, and many people might say, buy stock or crypto and leave it for years. The question is, does that suit your plan? Or do you want to invest in a seasonal crop in agriculture and get your profit in three or six months? You have to be clear about your financial plans. Remember, none of these vehicles is better than the other. Your plan will determine which is right for you. If you don't have a plan, don't bother to invest.

TRADING IS NOT INVESTING

Too many people focus on the product, let's say crypto currency, and the procedure, trading, but they don't have a plan. So, they can find themselves in the same circle for so long and never get ahead financially. Many people are trying to make money but what they think about investment is not the same as an investment but an act of trading.

Trading is a procedure or technique. Buying a crypto currency when it's low and selling when its high is not much different than a person who buys a house, fixes it up, and sells it for a higher price: one trade crypto, other trade real estate. Too many people get attached to one investment vehicle and don't see the opportunity in other vehicles. They think their vehicle is the best. When they get attached, they get to focus on the vehicle more than the plan. They make a lot of money buying, holding, and selling investment products that money may not take them to where they want to be financial. A true investor doesn't become attached to the vehicle or a procedure. A true investor wants to get from where they are financial to where they want to be within the desired time.

On the journey of making your dream a reality, you want to be smart about the investment vehicle you pick; you want to ensure it will return your profit to you within the desired time. If you plan on writing a book for six months or a year before you start editing and proofreading and all other essentials, you want to be sure your investment vehicle will yield profit back in 5month or 11 months. You don't want to buy a crypto currency and pray it will yield profit in 5 or 11 months, you have to be clear about how much profit you will make, and the time you will get the money back before your investment. You should know what happens if the investment goes well and what happens if the investment goes badly. Write a plan with a time frame to execute, don't forget we are talking about investing in financing your dreams.

INVESTMENT IS NOT RISKY:

Investing is not risky, not being finance literate is what is risky. The more you grow in knowledge financially, the more you can recognize the right or wrong investments for you. If you are going to become financially successful, you need to be a financial literate. It's not a one-time job; you have to keep learning for life if you want to be ahead financially. Imagine someone that makes 10 million dollars annually for five years; if the person doesn't upgrade their knowledge financially, they might get struck at 10 million dollars and soon start making less than 10 million dollars. The level of your income reflects the level of your knowledge about finance. When your mind has the information you need, making money becomes automatic. Making money becomes a lifestyle.

If you want to be a doctor, you'll go to medical school. If you want to be a lawyer, you'll go to law school to study law. If you want to be able to manage investment risk, then you have to study investment. How? Get financial advisers or mentors and coaches to produce the result you want. The world is at our fingertips today, but pick your investment vehicle and research it online. I bet; as you research, you will find ads, courses, and mentors that can help you get through. You can decide to check one or more people to compare before picking who you would like to educate you.

Investing is not risky; it's you who stands at risk if you are not financially educated.

THE MAGIC OF COMPOUNDING

Albert Einstein was amazed at how money could multiply just by the power of compounding. He considered the compounding of money to be one of the most amazing inventions. He said, "Compound interest is the 8th wonder of the world. Those who understand it earn it, those who don't pay for it."

Compounding is the process in which an asset's earnings, from either capital gains or interest are reinvested to generate additional earnings over time. Compounding, therefore, differs from linear growth, where only the principal earns interest each period, this requires patience, and the result is seen down the road; this is how many wealthy people have built their wealth over time. It's not about the money you're investing but how much time you allow it to grow. Young people are at a significant advantage in allowing their money to grow.

Warren Buffet is one of the best investors in the world. Read what he says about compounding, "My wealth has come from a combination of living in America, some lucky genes, and compound interest."

The bank used to be an excellent way to compound your money, but not anymore today. Many vehicles are great for compounding money today. If you are in your teenage years and twenties, you are at an advantage in compounding money, which results in financial freedom. So, I would recommend the book "The Compounding Effect" by Darren Hardy. If you are going to become successful, compounding has to become your habit. If you don't like reading books, get audiobooks.

IDEA:

It doesn't take money to make money.

Having an idea doesn't translate to being successful. It's what you do with the idea that makes you successful. Almost everyone has an idea, and many are still poor. Why? They are not executing the idea. Some execute but don't know how to monetize the idea. Having an idea is not enough to become successful. Maybe you don't have any source of income presently; you don't have any money to invest in yourself or money to multiply money. That's a great start; don't be discouraged because the truth is, it doesn't take money to make money. It takes your mind and plan.

If you have the opportunity to meet your younger self, what will you tell you to avoid mistakes? Imagine someone gave you materials on things to do and not do to avoid the mistakes you made. Will you be willing to pay for such material to get ahead faster in all ramifications of life? I bet many people will say yes. Now, imagine, you get the privilege to teach people that were once you how to avoid the mistakes you made and teach them how to get ahead faster. How cool will that be? People out there need your story to find hope. Many needs to hear you share your story of how you survived what they are going through presently, and this will give them courage. What problem can you solve right now; what can you do, and you know you're good at it that others will pay you.

On a lovely Saturday afternoon, I called a sister of mine, and we spoke about finance. Months before this call, I told her to read the first series of the book rich dad poor dad. After reading, she said to me. ''I didn't even know I was shaming money. I didn't realize how my poverty mindset was preventing me from having a good relationship with money'' **At that moment, I remembered how opportunities surrounded me, but couldn't see them because I had not trained my mind**.

If you plan to start your financial journey or you are on your financial journey, another book you want to pick up is "Rich dad poor dad."

As the discussion continued, she said, I called my cousin and told her we need to get back to making lamps. I asked what she meant by lamps. She explained; a lamp that lights up the room at night like a side light. It looks like an award but is made with glass. Words are engraved on the glass with silver glitters. She sent the picture to me so I could understand what she was saying. The first thing that came out of my mouth was, what in the world have you been doing and not selling this beautiful lamp?

I ask you again, what can you help others with that they will pay you for? Betty! I don't think this will work. If you say so, that will eventually become your reality. It doesn't take money to make money. It takes your mind and a plan. Making money is 80% psychology and 20%skills. Your words become your reality. What can you do that can help others become better? What are you good at? Without a doubt, you deliver immediately without preparation?

List 5 things that comes to your mind.

....

....

....

....

....

If nothing is coming, ask yourself repeatedly until you get an answer.

SELLING:

Earlier I asked you if someone gave you a manual to avoid mistakes and get ahead faster, would you pay for it. I bet you'll say yes. You paid for this book, most likely online. Imagine the person who created the platform where we both transact is still in doubt if people will like it. Asking question like

''Will I make money from it''

''There are people doing what I want to do.''

Just imagine that person is struck with the ideas in his/her head, then you and I might not find our transaction as smooth as we did. Imagine there is no online banking, every time you have to withdraw, you have to go to banks and stand for long hours. Online banking was once an idea in someone's head. Imagine the person was so scared to work on the idea because he's lost on who will like the idea.

An idea pops up in your head because there is someone out there who needs that solution. God placed that idea in your heart because he knows you can deliver. Have you had any idea before, and you stay in your head too long asking what people will say until you find someone who has that same idea and making money from it? Imagine you went to the mall to get your groceries for the week, and there were no goods in the mall because all the farmers and producers are stuck in their heads, saying, "Who will buy from us?"

What I'm trying to say is that every time you have an opportunity to make another person's life better and you don't sell to them because you're stuck in your head, you are doing them a disservice. You're robbing them of the chance to be a better person. Focus not on you but on the result another human being will have because you choose to serve them through your knowledge.

If only you were aware of what you can do, no one would know you can help them. You have to come out of hiding and let people around you know you are good at this and can help them through it. Your gifts are normal to you that you think it's easy for others as it is easy for you.

The more people you serve, the more money you make. Marketing is the oxygen for every successful business; marketing is attracting those who you can help with your product. Betty, this might take a while. Well, to go faster, pay mentors; Pay those who are getting the result you want to teach you

GET A JOB:

Don't forget that you are still in the chapter to fund your dreams. The goal is to fund your dream. On the journey to fund your dream, you need to be financially secure. When you are secure, you can move to comfortable and then rich. The truth is, some don't even want to become rich. They want to be comfortable; they want to be able to afford their basic needs and something they desire. Some want to stop being secured, living to meet up with their basic needs.

To make your dreams a reality, you have to be secured. Being secured means you have the basic needs; a house with running water and light to live in. and food to eat.

On the journey to make your dreams a reality. It's essential to be secured first. To be secured, get a job with your plan at the back of your mind. How long do I have to work?

How much do I need to save from this job before I quit?

You are back to plan again.

If you are getting a job, what's your plan? At some point, you might think of having to get a second job but while working at a job, start working out your dream instead of getting a second job.

You might need to start a business. You don't have to start a business because you like it, but, because you need it to fund your dream. Many great companies today start on a part-time basis. Michael Dell started his part-time business in his dorm room as a freshman at the University of Texas, Austin. He took orders over the phone, and before you know it, the sales skyrocketed, making it one of the fastest-growing companies ever. He had to quit school because his part-time business was making him far more prosperous than any course he was studying could pay. He never stopped learning. Five years into his business adventure, he took business classes at Stanford.

We are stubborn on vision, we are flexible on details, and we don't give up on things quickly. Our third-party seller business is an example of that. It took us three attempts to get the third-party seller business to work, and we didn't give up. If you're not stubborn, you'll give up on experiments too soon, and if you're not flexible, you'll pound your head against the wall, and you won't see a different solution to a problem you're trying to solve." - Jeff Bezos.

Jeff Bezos is the founder of Amazon, the world's largest online retailer. At 30 years, Bezos started this part-time job in his garage. He started with just books. In 1994, he quit his job.

"We've had three big ideas at Amazon that we've stuck with for 18 years, and they're the reason we're successful: put the customers first. Invent and be patient."

In some cases, things are inevitable. The hard part is that you don't know how long it might take, but you know it will happen if you're patient enough. E-books had to happen. Infrastructure web services had to happen so you can do these things with conviction if you are long-term-oriented and patient – Jeff Bezos.

DIGITAL AGE:

The economic world you were born into no longer exists. From the 1st wave of wealth to the 2nd wave of wealth, those that became wealthy were those who saw the opportunity at the end of an era and took massive actions.

WALMART VS AMAZON:

Walmart is known as the world's largest retailer, but that changed when Forbes mentioned that Amazon had overtaken Walmart. Amazon started as an e-commerce retailer and is now the largest online retailer in the world. Amazon set up a shop as an online bookseller when buying anything from the internet was a radically new idea for many Americans, and two decades later, the company today became more valuable than Walmart.

If Amazon was trying to be competitive with Walmart, there is no way he would have made it through. But he saw the future of the internet and started selling books in 1994, making his first sales in July 1995. But he envisioned the future and what it could be; when he told his parent to invest in his company, he said, "My father asked me what the internet is.'' To tell you and remind you that your dreams are ahead. Work them out, don't change your plan but be flexible in your approach.

It's the same with Zappos shoes. In 1994, Nick Swinmurn founded Zappos and launched the company with Tony Hsieh and Alfred Lin. Tony later became the CEO and retired in 2020 before he died. Zappos started selling shoes online; funny enough, it's the same year Amazon started. Free shipping for people to test if the shoe is their size and free shipping back to Zappos from customers. For many years, he lost financially, and Tony was the only one who continued to invest in the business. He believes in customer experiences. Today, Zappos is known to provide the best customer service and customer experience. Two decades later, Jeff Bezos bought Zappos for $1.2 billion in 2009.

WHERE IS THE MONEY NOW?

We are in the third wave of wealth now, and the first person to create wealth is not Elon Musk. Elon Musk belongs to the 2nd wave of wealth. The first person to create Wealth was Sam Bank man Fried. He was featured on Forbes 2021 and recognized for $ 24 billion. He was frustrated by the Japanese bank that made it very difficult to buy bitcoin, so he decided to create a foreign exchange platform called FTX; this happened in 2019. However, he started crypto in 2017. At 29 years, he became a cryptocurrency billionaire and became the 32nd richest man in the world.

You can still partake in the wealth; you are not early, but not so late too. You can still get in.

The new oil is making money online. **Tai Lopez** said, "2020 ended the informative age. We are now on the rise of the sovereign nation." it has come to stay, and it's not going any time soon. You are in the new norm; you are never going back to the old ways. When the industrial age came, what went around was going to school and getting a good grade, and securing a good job. In the informative age, that doesn't work. Those that pivot by leveraging on the online business prove good to school as an old principle. Yet, many are still stuck in going to school to secure a job. You are in the era of learning skills and working from home. In this era, there is more money than ever. You make money at the level of self-education [get mentored, book reading, courses], not school education. You have to educate your mind to see the opportunities around you.

Ways to make money online: all these are done from the comfort of your home.

Cryptocurrency

Affiliate marketing

Social media marketing

Network marketing

Video editing

Content creator

Graphic design

Importation

Exportation

Drop shipping

Drop servicing

Forex

MONETIZE YOUR GIFT:

Every gift can be monetized. If you don't learn the business side of your gift, it will continue to be a hobby, and there are many people in your gift industry making millions. If you don't learn the business side, you will have to get another source of income to meet your basic needs. How great is it if you do what you love so much and get paid for it? Imagine what life would be. You can live on your gift if you learn to monetize it.

I listened to Steve Harvey as he talked about his barber. He said, the first time he barbed my hair was for $10. When he came to Steve Harvey's show, he barbed $1500 per haircut. Steve cut his hair 4times a month. That's $ 6000 in a month. **"He almost killed himself when I went bald,"** Steve said. Now! He got four salons in Texas and 2 Barber College and makes 6million dollars a year. Your dream will make room for you and make you sit among kings and queens when you have the mindset it takes to be in the room in the first place. If you don't display your gift, no one will know you have them.

Write a financial plan to fund your Dream? Your Dream might be short-term or long-term, and without a plan, you can't get ahead financially; you make money but won't be financially free.

How much do you want to make in the next six months, one year..........continue with "clarity questions" from chapter 3.

CHAPTER 6

DIE EMPTY

You are the designer of your destiny, you are the author of your story. —Lisa Nichols

When I hear people say the quote above, the old version of me cringes and try to fight on God's behalf. How in the world will someone say they are the designer of their destiny, the author of their story? What do you mean by that? Where do you put God? I would silently ask myself. As I study more, I realize God is in partnership with us. If He's going to do anything for us and through us, we have to partner with Him, without your partnership God can't do anything through you and with you. If He does, that against the willpower he gave you. God is not in the business of going against your willpower or forcing you to do anything. Not even the devil can force you to do anything you don't want to do. However, he's good at manipulating the mind so you can submit your will subconsciously, and he then acts. The devil really can't do anything without your permission.

God chooses your destiny, but you decide if you'll partner with Him to make that destiny a reality. You have a role to play, and God has a role to play to birth your destiny. God has purposed it, but you must create it here on earth. He chose it, and you have to make it a reality as He directs your path. It's your responsibility to make it a reality. If you do not partner with Him, that which He wants to make a reality through you won't happen. Even though God has chosen and commanded our destinies, you decide to create it here on earth. So, you are the designer of your destiny, the author of your story.

YOUR LIFE IS YOUR RESPONSIBILITY:

No one is coming to rescue you, you're your rescue. - Lisa Nichols.

You need to give yourself permission to live the life of your dream. You need to give the greatness inside of you permission to come forth. You need to be willing to rescue your future and protect your future memory. You need to be you. You are better when you are your authentic self. Your life is your responsibility. No one can design your life better than you. No one can write your story like you, you are the author of your autobiography, and no one, I repeat, no one can help you than you.

You wait for permission from your spouse, friends, family, and colleagues to approve the vision that God shared with you. How do you expect them to understand the vision God shared with you and not them? How do you expect them to be excited and come aligned with the vision? Some might understand you the first time you talk about it, and that's great if they do. You might have to communicate your vision with your loved ones over and over again before they understand you. Don't get mad if they don't understand the first time. It's your vision, not theirs? But your conviction expressed through tenacity and action can convince them. When they see you taking actions, it's easier for them to give you their permission.

You should understand that you need to give yourself permission first before anyone else. If you don't give yourself permission, it won't be easy for your spouse, friends, and colleagues to give you their permission.

While you're waiting on God, God is waiting on you. You pray for financial breakthroughs, business idea pops up in your head. You didn't plan towards the idea, research on things you need to make it a reality, and you continue to pray. It's your responsibility and not God's to plan on how to execute that vision. It's your responsibility to learn the skills and capability to make that vision a reality. You have to ensure you gain the right mindset to execute the vision God has shared with you. When God shares a vision with you, and you don't have the mindset for it, you use words like,

"I'm not enough," "I don't think I'm qualified," "This is too good for me," "I can't do it." For these reasons, many have lost the blessing God had for them. They failed to upgrade their mindset and realize the idea was the answer to their prayer.

God is a gracious God. He look for ways to get your mind to understand the vision he has shared with you. If your mind doesn't get it, you can't execute. You might have a challenge that will result in changing your mindset. You can come across a book that will enlighten your mind in that area, a friend can come to speak to you in that area, and you can find a relevant video that will help you. This is why it is said, "Life happens for us, not to us." When you have this mindset, you can ask, what is this situation trying to teach me, not make a statement like, "Why is this happening to me." or "I'm always a victim." The blessing is delayed, not because God is not ready, but because you are not ready. Your spirit, soul, and body must be involved to birth a vision. Your spirit receives the information, your mind interprets what your spirit has received. If your mind doesn't understand, you don't understand either. How do you execute what you don't understand? When your body gets the information from your soul, you'll find out that you'll wake up without an alarm clock to do what you have to do.

You have been praying, and your situation has not changed. You might say it's not the right time, or you are waiting on God. What if God is waiting on you to have the skills and capability? What if God is waiting on you to have the right mindset? What if God is waiting on you to immerse yourself in the right knowledge? What if God is waiting on you to take the first step so He can show you the next step?

In Hosea 4:6 book of the Holy Bible, God says, "My people are destroyed for the lack of knowledge." God didn't say my people are destroyed because they can't pray or don't have power. He said they are dying of a lack of knowledge. When you
Read that verse further, God said, "I have rejected them and won't allow them to represent me."

God doesn't want ignorant people to represent Him. I was surprised when I realized this fact. Can it be you are in your present situation because you're waiting on God while God is waiting on you?

I was speaking with a friend of mine. In the conversation, she said, "I'm just waiting on God to tell me what to do next" this was after she had received the vision. I said can I tell you something? God has permitted you. It's your turn to permit yourself. When you receive a vision and you're convinced you are meant to do it, it's time to learn the skills and capability essential for it. Are you waiting on God's permission while God is waiting on your action?

GREATNESS IS IN YOU:

Stop thinking you will wake up one day and find yourself in greatness and everything will work out fine. Success is a journey. You have to work it out; you grow into greatness. Only you can work out the result you want for your life. Your loved ones have a limit to which they can help you. The day you realize your life is your responsibility and that if you don't get up and take massive actions towards what you want, you won't have them is the day you truly start living. If you want to change your life, you have to change. If you want things to be different, you have to be different. If you want things to be better, you have to be better. Every day, you have the privilege to design your life the way you want it. The life you want is on the other side of inconvenient. you know you can do better than you do. You know there are things you're good at, you know you have greatness inside of you, but you must be willing to birth it at all costs. Many destinies are tied to yours; you getting up will provoke other destinies to get up.

DESTINY IS WAITING ON YOU TO GET UP

The wealthiest place on the planet earth is the graveyard. In the cemetery are books never written, music that no one has ever heard, paints no one has ever seen, poetry no one ever seen nor heard. It's filled with businesses that never opened, ideas that never came to fruition, and dreams that never came to reality. It's so full of wealthy and great men who died as alcoholics, great women who died as prostitutes, and so on. Myles Munroe.

You and I are candidates to add to the cemetery. We have a decision to make daily not to make the graveyard rich. We have a decision to bring to reality the pictures God keeps showing us over and over again. Those pictures are real. Many destinies need to see you birth those pictures for them to get up and birth theirs. I appeal to you, don't add to the wealth in the graveyard, those pictures in your head since childhood, the imaginations you can't let go of are real, make them real. Destinies are waiting to be impacted by the existence of your vision.

Your children need to see you execute them. Your family and spouse need to see you, your colleagues need to see you, and your circles need to see you execute them. Don't rob us of the gift of your contributions here on earth. Your contribution is essential. Your contribution makes everyone you come across better. You will always have a vision to execute. When you're done, you will know you will be able to say, **"I have done all that destiny required of me. If you're not, you will be scared of death".** **Myles Munroe**

Albert Einstein suffered a ruptured aneurysm, and he refused surgical treatment saying, "I want to go when I want. It is tasteless to prolong life artificially. I have done my share; it is time to go. I will do it elegantly."

POTENTIAL:
The wealth in the cemetery can be referred to as potential. Potential is who you can be, but you are not yet. It's a hidden strength, currently unrealized ability, undeveloped ability, untapped power, dormant ability. Potential is never what you've done. When you've done something, it's no longer your potential. That's why you should never be proud of what you've done. It's simply behind you and is no longer your potential.

God is glad you unleash the last potential but more eager to see you unleash the potential for this season. Every manufacturer is glad to see their products work in the way they've been programmed. It's the same with God. It excites him to watch you unleash your potential per season and not get stuck with the things you did last season. The last vision is gone. What's the new vision, and which part of you need to unfold to execute this new vision? The cemetery is filled with potential because they never manifest the extraordinary abilities, gift, and talents that God hide in each of them.

SEED:

Fact is collected information that can be arrived at by logical conclusion and can be mere statistical data. **Truth** is the validity of collected facts, they are not arrived at by logical conclusions. Truth has to be either seen or experienced to prove its validity. Truth is universal. Facts are not universal. Truth is the same anywhere in the world, but the same can't be said for a fact.

If I hold a seed of apple and ask you what's in my hand, you would reply seed. That's the fact. The truth is, I have an apple tree. But, that's not the complete truth because the apple tree will grow apple fruit that has a seed, and that seed is the potential of another apple tree, and the circle continues. The truth of what's in my hand is a forest, not a seed. Inside, every little boy is an extraordinary man. Every little girl is a powerful woman. In every failure, God hides success.

The potential inside of you are seeds that can become a forest when unleashed. Your seed can result in an unrecognizable future if you give it permission to grow, your seed can result in financial freedom if you give it permission. Your seed can make you stand before kings if you learn the skills and capability to be excellent at it.

It's quite easy to ignore a seed than a forest, it's easier to destroy a seed than a forest, that's why it seems there are so many things to distract you. You have a seed, and you can't see the forest of what your seed can become. Therefore, you speak ill of yourself. Sometimes, you think it's easier to give up. It's not about now but the result of what you carry.

YOU ARE OF GREAT WORTH:
No matter how dysfunctional your background, how broke or broken you are, where you are today, or what anyone says, you MATTER, and your life matters. –Germany Kent

To have whatever you want, you have to believe you are worthy of it. If you have something and you feel you are not worthy of it, it's only a matter of time. You will lose it. Your mind will fight it till you lose it. I want you to know that you are worthy of a good spouse. You are worthy of financial freedom. You are worthy of people that love your vibe and show up for you. You are worthy of great things. You deserve them. Every morning, learn to convince yourself that you're worthy of a good life. You are worthy of abundant life. You are worthy of manifesting the life you constantly dream about. Wake up courageously every day to make your dream life a reality. Until you realize and accept your worthy of your dream life, you can't have the life you want.

DON'T LET YOUR CIRCUMSTANCE HOLD YOU BACK.

A young boy was born in Marlboro, New York; at age 3, his parent divorced, and he had to stay with his mom and grandma. He switched between his mom and dad severally till he was 19. He watches as both parents struggle financially. He decided he was not going to live his life that way. He had difficulties in school. In the adulthood stage, he found out his difficulty in school was because he had dyslexia. He completed high school and never had the opportunity to go to college. He worked with his father in his car repair shop. He began to repair, purchase and re-sell cars. He also got into real estate. Though he had no capital but made a smart move by buying a run-down apartment without putting any money down. He made a lot of money.

He was hungry for more and wanted to teach people but didn't know how. Fortunate for him, he came across Tony Robbins infomercials, which he bought and provided him with the information he needed. That was how the young man was able to achieve his first real success in his twenties. While in his twenties, he got a house for both parents and changed their cars every 2years. The young boy then is whom we know as Dean Graziosi.

Today, Dean Graziosi is known as an iconic entrepreneur, a successful marketer, a successful coach, and the author of 5 bestselling books. Presently, he works on a project with Tony Robbins called mastermind, which has transformed almost 50,000 people's life by introducing them to the self-education industry.

Dean is currently selling a book, "Millionaire Success Habits" he has sold over 1 million copies. Dean is phenomenal. You need to hear him speak, and you will testify. What most people say about Dean is his passion for helping people as much as he can.

What's your story? Dean has dyslexia. He couldn't read or write. He experienced childhood trauma but was determined to live a different from his parent. He didn't go to college but succeeded through self-education.

What story are you telling yourself that's holding you back from success? Maybe you are saying, "My parent didn't provide all I needed to have a successful life." Dean didn't have that either. He rose against all odds. You should stop the pity story and start telling yourself the right story. If Dean could rise against all odds, then you can. Your circumstances don't determine your future; your background doesn't determine your future. Your decisions determines your future. You determine what your future will look like. It's in your hands. God won't fail in directing you, but you have to believe in your future. You have to create the future you want and make the imaginations in your head a reality. It's your responsibility.

You don't need all you think you need. What you need to start with is what you have now! What's your future going to be like? You determine that, not God.

KEEP TRYING TILL YOU GET IT RIGHT:

Every time I see a flying plane, I'm continually intrigued by how a plane would fly from the ground up and come back down when it gets to its destination. Many people have heard about the Wright brothers, Wilbur and Orville. The question is, what inspired them?

When they were young, their father got them a helicopter toy which stirred their love for aeronautics. The Wright brothers were in the printing and bicycle business before they went entirely into aeronautics. Their knowledge of both businesses helped in their aeronautics journey. They both began by studying aeronautic books and closely followed the research of German aviator Otto Lilienthal. In their study of designs and accomplishments of others, they realized no one had found a way to control the aircraft while in the air. With their determination to succeed, they move to "Kitty Hawk" North Caroline for its strong wind, hills, and sands for a soft landing. They study how the birds fly and how the birds angled their wings for balance and control, and they emulate it.

December 17, 1903, they succeeded in flying the first airplane after many failed trials and building their engine themselves alongside Charles Taylor. Wilbur flew their plane for 59 seconds over a distance of 852feet. It was an outstanding achievement. The Wright brothers soon discovered those around them did not appreciate their efforts; the media, and fellow flight experts. They made a move from America to Europe in 1908 to convince the public and sell airplanes, and they succeeded. The Wright brothers succeeded in France. They were hosted by royals and heads of state and were constantly featured by the press. They became celebrities, sold some airplanes, got contracts, and became wealthy businessmen before returning to the United States.

So many odds stand against the Wright brothers, but they rose above the odds of who are we to make an aircraft that would fly. They could have told themselves. We don't have college degrees, we don't have money, and we are not in the location to help with a soft landing. In achieving your dream, many odds will stand in your way. Are you willing to overcome all odds?

Are you willing to be okay if people around act like they don't see your success at first?

Are you willing to change location and environment to suit your dreams?

Are you willing to give all for your dream?

THE BEST INVESTMENT YOU CAN MAKE IS IN YOURSELF:

A young boy born and raised in America at 17years has watched how his mother re-married severally and how they don't have enough money to eat. He grew up in a chaotic and abusive home. He was working as a janitor but needed extra cash. A man his parents knew and whom his father had called a "loser" had become quite successful in a short time, at least in financial terms. He was buying, fixing, and flipping real estate in Southern California and needed a kid on the weekend to help him move furniture.

One weekend while the young boy was working his tail off, it led to an opening that changed his life forever. The young boy had a moment with the rich man, and he asked him, "How did you turn your life around? The rich man replied, "By going to a seminar by a man named Jim Rohn." "What's a seminar?" he asked. "It's a place where a man takes ten or twenty years of his life and all he's learned, and he condenses it into a few hours so that you can compress years of learning into days," he answered. Wow, that sounded pretty awesome. "How much does it cost?" "Thirty-five dollars," he told me. What! The young buy was making **$40 a week** as a part-time janitor while going to high school. "Can you get me in?" he asked the rich man, sure, but you wouldn't value it if you don't pay for it.'

The young boy won the battle in his mind and paid for the seminar. He went again and again. He began to read books and buy tapes. He went to get more jobs to sustain him while all this was going on. He was living in a car, and his mom threw him out the same day with his stepfather because he was speaking on his behalf.

The young boy attends Jim Rohn's seminar repeatedly, to be mentored by him. This would cost him $12000. There was no hope of where a poor boy could get that amount, but the conviction of his dream made him find a way to get the money. He went straight to the bank and asked the bank for a loan. He had no property to put down, and he was not 18 years yet. All force seemed to be against him. He stood by the cashier and said, "I would pay back." I need this money to help change my life so I can change many people's life. He stayed by the cashier for a long time.

The cashier said the bank couldn't borrow him the money, but she will. "I have never seen a young boy so convinced about his dream as you. I will lend you the money, but you have to pay it back." He said thank you, I will. He replied to the cashier. The woman asked for a postal address, He has no address because he lives in a car. The cashier lends him the money. That young boy is **Tony Robbins.**

Tony Robbins has truly empowered more than 50 million people from 100 countries around the world through his audio programs, educational videos, and live seminars. He's an author of 6 best-selling books, a philanthropist, and the nation's #1 life and business strategist. Tony feeds a million American yearly. He's involved in more than 100 privately held businesses with combined sales exceeding $ 7 billion a year. He has worked with 4 American presidents and many celebrities across the industries.

Tony Robbins could have struggled and allowed his mind to win the battle of spending all the $40 weekly pay on food, but he invested in himself. The best investment you can ever make is to invest in yourself. Jim Rohn said, **"Work hard on yourself than you do on your job."** When you increase in value, your income also increases. Tony could have given up on how to get the $12000, He was a 17years old from a poor family and later kicked out of the house. His conviction about his dream was all over him, and the banker decided to borrow him.

I ask you again;

Are you willing to pay the price for your dream life?

Are you willing to be certain and overcome all obstacles?

Are you willing to let go of the latest designers to have an unrecognizable future?

Are you willing to invest a large amount of your income in your future?

Are you willing to be inconvenient now for the future you want?

YOU WILL WIN IF YOU DON'T QUIT:

Mrs. Folorunsho Alakija is a Nigeria billionaire oil tycoon, a fashion designer, a real estate manager, and a philanthropist. She is known to have displaced Oprah Winfrey as the richest black woman in the world. This changed in 2021 due to a pandemic affecting the oil demand.

The majority of her wealth is from her oil business. It took her 3years to gain the oil license. She had to visit the petroleum minister three times before she got the license, and each appointment took her six months or more to process. Most time, she had to start all over again due to a change in the petroleum minister. Instead of being frustrated, she told herself she would get to the bottom of this. I don't give up easily, she said to herself. As every door is about to open, she meets a new petroleum minister and have to start the process all over again.

Finally, she was handed land that was 5000 feet deep in water. It was terrible enough exploring on land and now on water that technology has not reached. It was expensive to explore, and she couldn't fund it. She had to look for technical partners. The first she found, when they saw where the land is, they declined, same with the second technical partner. But she didn't give up. She said to herself that she would go around to many companies. I have nothing to lose, she said. While all this was going on, she was a success in the fashion industry.

It took her three years to get technical partners and another three months to negotiate and conclude. These partners are entitled to 40% of the income. Put in mind that this is a block nobody wanted. In fact, those who once got the block returned it. One day, the technical partner reached out and said they had struck oil in commercial quantity. Exploring is expensive if it's not in commercial quantity there is no need for further digging, she said

Then, the government came in to take 50% from the 60% left with Mrs. Alakija after she gave her partner 40%. The government was concerned that after tax and other expenses, the oil company stood a chance of making 10 million dollars a day. She took the government to court, and this went on for 12 year, and she won the case. She said even before she got the license. She was observing 40 days fast, one after the other.

I'm asking you again, are you willing to fight for your dreams? Are you willing to go all in for what you want? Are you willing to pay the price for what you want? Mrs. Alakija could have given up within the first three years of trying to gain a license or when she found out nobody wanted the oil block that was given to her and when the government said they wanted 50% from her 60%. She fought the government for twelve years. Her conviction made her pull through. Are you convinced about your dream? How long can you fight for your dream? Are you willing to fight for 12 years if it's going to take you that long?

Are you willing to overcome the obstacles on your way to achieving your dream? Are you willing to be inconvenient? Are you willing to look crazy to those around you to get what you want? Are you willing to play full out? Are you willing to fight till you see the pictures in your head become a reality?

Are you willing to take full responsibility for your life?
Are you willing to pay the price of success?
Are you willing to be inconvenient for a while?
Are you willing to pay the price of focus?
Are you willing to be disciplined?
Are you willing to leave something behind?

Success is not cheap. Don't think life will bend success principles for you because you have prayed. After praying, you have to do the work. Mrs. Alakija prayed, did her research, and got educated in areas she needed to. Success won't fall on your lap because you have prayed, you have to do the work. Don't give up too soon. Your dream will cost you many things but will be worth it at the end of the day. If you hang in there, you'll win. Quitters never win. Winners never quit.

DIE EMPTY NOT EARLY:

Our lives have been predetermined, and you don't know the date you'll check out from here. But one thing is sure. You are predetermined to check out at a particular time, and this time, you are expected to have manifested all that your manufacturer expects from you. Regardless, you can haste to check out early from the choices you make, your lifestyle, the places you go, the people you move with, what you eat, what you listen to and watch, staying in an abusive environment, the others abound.

One of the tools you need to implement your assignment is your body. Once it's not healthy, implementing your assignment will be hindered. Prevent yourself from anything and anyone that could cause you to die early.

The goal is not to die early but die empty. By the time you have come to the last days of your life, you'll look at the roles you've played, and you'll should be excited. At the end of your life, you don't want to tell yourself, I wish I didn't give up on the business, my dreams. I wish I had tried the fifth business, it might have turned out to be a success. No! The story you want to tell yourself is I gave my all. I gave everything I had. You don't want to add to the graveyard's wealth but subtract. The reason you have to protect your memory now. In your last days, you can have adventures, fun, and an excellent memory. **Live your life authentically and live it as the internal GPS guides you. Winners never quit. Quitters never win!**

ONE LAST MESSAGE

Congratulations!

I'm proud of you that you've completed this book. Many talk about achieving more in finance, leadership and life but take no action. I admire and respect you for wanting to improve your finance, leadership and life.

My mission with this book is to give you the mindset you need for success and own your future.

My hope is that you have become more inspired and empowered to be more, do more and achieve more.

Whether you achieve your dreams and goals is solely up to you. No one can promise or guarantee what level of success you will achieve.

However, by following simple success strategies like those in this book, you can begin to accomplish anything you desire.

YOU CAN DO IT – THE BEST TIME TO START IS NOW

Again, congratulations.

> **"Knowledge is not enough, massive action is what get you the result you desire."** *-Betty Olowokere*

Acknowledgments

My life has been impacted by many shared ideas, mentors and support, each in different ways. It's impossible to thank everyone and I apologies for anyone not listed. Please know that I appreciate you greatly.

First and foremost, I'm grateful for the privilege of being in a relationship with God. Special gratitude to my parent, Mr. Bayo and Mrs. Kehinde Olowokere; thank you for your investment in my life. Pastor Lekan Odewumi, and Owoyemi Oyinkansola, I appreciate your dedication to completing this book. Deenuka Nagrendra, Dean Graziosi, Tony Robbins, Lisa Nichols, James Malinchak, Nick Unsworth, Megan Unsworth, Mrs Bolaji Adesoba, Mrs Dolapo Momoh, Mrs Solape Olojede, Rev. Chris Oyakhilome, Prophet Abiodun Sule, Pastor Terry Yakubu Ishaku, Pastor Tosin Amusan, Dr. Priscilla Ajetumobi, Mrs Folorunsho Alakija, Mrs Funke Felix Adejumo, Mrs Olajumoke Adenowo, Pastor Laju Iren. Bishop T.d Jakes, Sarah Jakes Roberts. Catherine Akapo, Doyinsola Esther, Cindy Trim, Juanita Bynum.

ABOUT BETTY

Betty Olowokere is an Author, life coach and doctor in

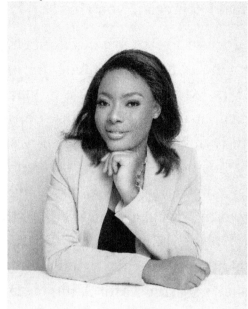

training. Her mission for the past seven years has been to teach people how to unleash their potential and become their best version. She has mentored many on how to build and grow in relationships with God.

Betty is passionate and committed to serving people at the highest level possible. She helps people realize that their dream life is possible and that it all starts with a mindset.

Contact

www.bettyolowokere.com
Email: betty@bettyolowokere.com

REVIEW

You help get this book into the hand of others by sharing your review on the platform you got the book.
You can also send your review to

Contact

www.bettyolowokere.com
Email:Review@bettyolowokere.com

Special <u>FREE</u> Bonus Gift for You

To help you to achieve more success, there are
FREE BONUS RESOURCES for you at:

www.FreeGiftFromBetty.com

- Training video on how successful people and top achievers attract more opportunities, achieve more goals and own their future.

Printed in Great Britain
by Amazon

23014131R00106